MW01593707

TEACHING YOGA
BEYOND THE POSES

A Practical Workbook for Integrating Themes, Ideas, and
Inspiration into Your Class, Dream Yoga, Rise & Shine Yoga
Flows, Yoga for a Healthy Mind and Body, Osteoporosis

By stephens donna adriene bible mark

Table of Contents

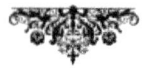

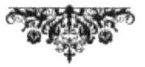

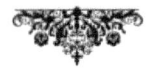

INTRODUCTION

Millions of people today are turning to Yoga to help them stay healthy and fit. Many people enjoy Yoga as a stress reliever after a hard day at the office. The popular belief is that Yoga is all about bending and twisting your body this way and that, likely ending up in your chiropractor's office. Many do not realize however, the full medicinal effects of Yoga and how it can improve their overall well-being.

Today Yoga is usually taught using the traditional methods and techniques of Hinduism. In fact Yoga itself derives many of its practices and ethics from the Hindu doctrine including their moral and ethical principles and spiritual philosophies. Contemplative meditation is also a practice they share.

Practitioners of Yoga view it as beneficial in their physical lives because it leads to improved health, mental focus, and intuitive well-being. The teachings of Yoga have transcended borders and religions and can be found all across the world. In Hinduism, practicing Yoga is looked

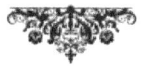

at as a practice to bring the practitioner closer to his or her deity. In Buddhists on the other hand, do not believe in a centralized deity. Still the practice of Yoga is prevalent among the Buddhist faith as a source of meditation and internal contemplation.

Yoga can help anyone become a mast of his or her body, mind and emotional well-being. People have said that Yoga is the way of increasing a spiritual understanding with the world around us, gaining the knowledge of the true nature of things. While studies have proven Yoga to be descended from a Hindu religious act, modern Yoga is not religious and is enjoyed by people of all nationalities and faiths.

Yoga techniques, texts and stories have traditionally been passed down from teacher to student for hundreds of years. With the advent of the Internet however, information about Yoga, its history, and its current practices are just a click away.

Yoga throughout history has helped its practitioners become more in tune with their physical and emotional

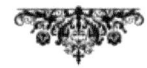

states and has contributed to the emergence of a new and
healthier culture in our country.

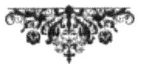

CHAPTER 1

HOW TO TEACH YOGA STUDENTS NEW POSES

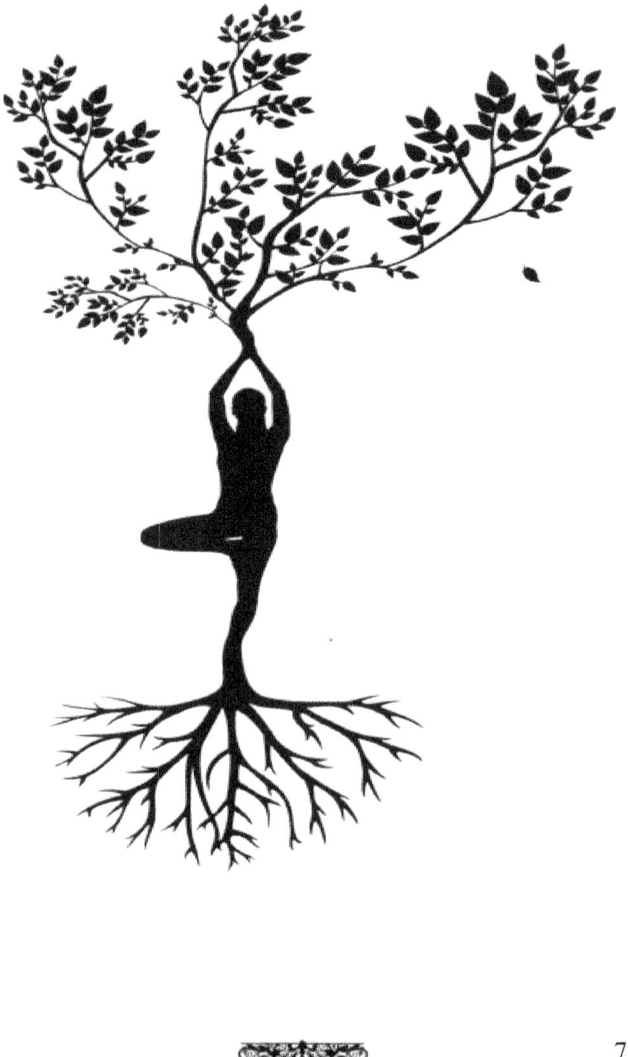

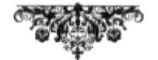

Yoga instructors who are interested in learning and growing with respect to their teaching capacities should know that teaching yoga students new poses can help them accomplish this objective. Instructors who are interested in learning how to teach yoga students new poses should know that there are several simple strategies they can implement to do so.

Here are four:

1. Practice Them Yourself.

In many cases, yoga instructors seek to teach yoga students new poses that have just become popular. When this happens, the yoga instructors themselves are not particularly familiar with the moves. For this reason, yoga instructors should practice new poses on their own before showing them to students. To make the most of this strategy, the instructor should practice the new yoga poses in front of a mirror. In so doing, he or she will be able to observe their own form and take any errors or structural deviations into account. Once instructors can execute a new pose without error, they will be ready to teach the move to students.

2. Show And Tell.

Typically, yoga instructors make one of two mistakes when they are attempting to teach yoga students new poses. They either "show" the students or "tell" the students. In the case of just showing, the yoga instructor does not give verbal instructions but simply executes the movement such that students learn by watching. Although this strategy can work for some students, it is not effective for every student. Why? Because many yoga students are auditory learners, meaning that their ability to grasp new material is highly contingent upon instructions and information being presented in a verbal format.

In the cases when a yoga instructor opts to simply "tell" students how to do a new pose, the rate of error and confusion will likely be high. This is the case because many yoga students are not auditory learners. Rather, they are visual and/or kinesthetic learners, meaning they need to see the movement executed or mimic the movements they've seen in order to master the move. In recognizing this, yoga instructors who want to maximize the likelihood that their students will master new moves should both show and tell their students what to do. This means that they should do a combination of the aforementioned teaching styles. By offering verbal

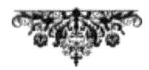

9

instructions and demonstrating the moves, people will be able to master the new poses irrespective of their learning style.

3. Watch, Watch, Watch.

As many fitness professionals know, yoga instructors have a tendency to become so immersed in mastering new poses and showing them to students that they forget the importance of carefully monitoring the students as they execute the moves. Yet this is an immensely important component of the teaching process. Why? Because by carefully watching students as they execute the movements, yoga instructors can detect and subsequently correct any errors that they make.

4. Offer Gentle Correction.

Throughout the process of teaching yoga students new moves, instructors will note that some of the students are performing the poses incorrectly. When this happens, the correct mode of action will be to provide gentle correction. This means avoiding the use of potentially harsh-sounding words like "No" or "Don't." It also means to compliment the student regarding anything they're doing correctly so that they will not dwell on their

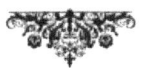

10

shortcomings. When yoga instructors offer gentle correction in this way, students are likely to maintain their confidence and self-esteem as they strive for improvement.

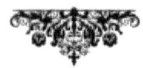

CHAPTER 2

HELPFUL STRATEGIES ON HOW TO TEACH YOGA CLASSES

Yoga is a type of exercise that takes a holistic approach to promoting mental, physical and spiritual health. It's an ancient practice which originated in India, although some forms of yoga were practiced in Egypt, China and other parts of the world as well. All told, this form of meditation dates back over five thousand years. Practitioners gain increased flexibility, balance and posture. Yet, this series of postures, poses and movements can also induce an healthy lifestyle. If you learn how to teach yoga classes, you can improve a person's life in many tangible ways.

If you want to teach classes, then first you need to determine which type of yoga you'll be teaching. There are subtle differences and you need to advise your prospective students about them. Bikram yoga, or hot yoga takes place in sauna-like conditions and focuses on body alignment. Kundalini yoga deals with the root chakra and is targeted at strengthening the core muscle

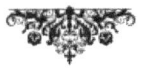

groups. Vinyasa yoga is all about movement and requires students to traverse seamlessly from one pose to another. These are just a few different types, but you should educate your students on which type of yoga you'll be teaching.

You need to determine a schedule for your classes. It's best to arrange them according to skill level. Group your beginners together, your intermediates and advanced students as well. This will ensure that everyone is progressing at their own pace and you can concentrate on individual needs within the class. Your class schedule should be sufficiently spread over the course of the week to give your students a chance to rest in-between sessions. You also need to consider your own physical and mental limitations. Don't make a demanding schedule that you can't maintain. As an instructor, you should perform at your best. Therefore, try to avoid scheduling your classes too close together.

Different people have different expectations, so you should have individual consultations with your students. If you aren't aware of previous injuries or health-related problems, then you could lead a student into a much worse

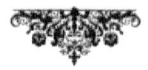

condition. Find out their expectations and limitations before you begin. You might not have to change your entire routine to accommodate a few students, but by having foreknowledge about their conditions, you can recommend alternate poses that will prevent them from worsening a nagging injury.

Lastly, take some time to think about the environment and the type of experience you want to provide. Yoga isn't just physical. It deals with mental focus, clarity of vision and an enhanced spiritual awareness. Your class should address these areas, but you have the creative freedom to approach this in a variety of different ways. Some instructors use colorful draperies and cushions to visually delight their practitioners. Other teachers might choose a selection of meditation tracks to create an auditory experience for their students. You can even suggest meals and snacks that take the yoga experience one step further. Be creative and look for ways to engage the student's on several different levels.

These are just a few things to consider before you start teaching classes. Ultimately, you'll have to trust your intuition. Yet, always stay focused on your primary goal,

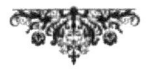

which is to enhance the lives of your student's through the wonders of yoga. The students will keep coming back to your class if they feel enriched and nurtured by the experience.

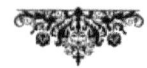

CHAPTER 3

HOW TO TEACH YOGA CLASSES FOR ALL ABILITY LEVELS

Teaching a yoga class is a big responsibility. You have to know how to get all of your students to relate to what you are teaching them despite everyone in your class having a different learning style as well as differing ability levels. What are some ways that you can learn how to teach yoga classes in an effective manner?

Pay attention during your own training classes

Before you start teaching your own classes, you will have to become a certified instructor. When you watch your teacher, look at what he or she does well and emulate that as best you can. In most cases, your teacher is going to be patient, charming and disarming of anything negative that happens during class. Think about whether or not you enjoyed your own learning experience and make sure that you make the learning experience fun for your students as well.

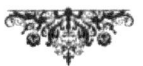

Listen to Your Students

Your students won't mind telling you whether you are doing a good job or not as an instructor. While they may not say that you are a bad teacher to your face, they will tell you how they feel by not showing up to your classes or using body language that suggests that they are not having a good time in your class. If you notice that your students are not coming back to class or don't seem to be interested in what is going on, you know that you need to change things up a bit.

Everyone is there to relax

The point of yoga is to relax and feel inner peace. This means that you need to be relaxed as well. Although it is easy to get excited when a class is going well or nervous when you first start teaching, you need to keep yourself calm or at least not let your emotions show through. However, the good news is that you shouldn't have a problem getting too high or too low as long as you were properly trained in the class that you are teaching.

Never Date Your Students

Just because your students may come to class in tight pants or other types of somewhat revealing clothing does not mean that you should hit on them or make any other

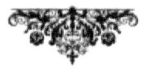

physical advances. Doing so could put the trust and confidence of a student in doubt and make you seem unprofessional. Over time, your students may see you as nothing more than a pickup artist who preys on those who pay good money to learn from you. While you can't control the actions of other people, you may want to strongly discourage students from dating other students or engaging in physical relationships outside of class.

Yoga is a great way to clear your mind and improve your fitness. If you are going to be a good yoga teacher, you need to be able to connect with your students in a meaningful and professional way. Therefore, remember to relax, keep the classes fun and never cross the line between student and teacher. This will ensure that you are successful in your teaching endeavor.

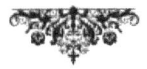

CHAPTER 4

LEARNING HOW TO TEACH YOGA STUDENTS

Over the past decade, yoga has emerged as one of the most popular forms of exercise. Going beyond a regular exercise program, yoga is a great way to learn meditation, relaxation and peace of mind. With so many yoga programs available, it can be difficult to make sure that your yoga studio stands out from the competition. The following guide provides effective tips on how to teach yoga students.

When teaching yoga students, it's important to create a calm, relaxing environment. Excessive noise and distractions should be minimized. If a yoga studio is located next to a noisy road, coffee shop or other location, it may be necessary to put up noise-blocking materials. Many online stores offer special soundproofing materials for walls. These materials can help mask the noises of the outside world.

Instead of outside noises, a yoga session should be accompanied by natural, healing sounds. Gentle, relaxing music is a great way to get students to let go completely.

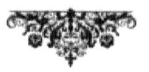

19

Scents can also be a great way to create a gentle, warm ambiance for a yoga session. Scents of lilac, rosewood and peppermint can help ensure a welcoming environment for all yoga students in your classroom.

When guiding students through each yoga pose, it's important to make sure that everyone feels welcome. Since most yoga classes comprise people of different skill levels, it's essential to offer poses that work for both beginners and advanced practitioners. For example, a basic downward dog pose will work well for people just learning about yoga. For advanced practitioners, a raised leg downward dog is a good choice. By providing different options for your students, everyone can work at his or her skill level.

Each yoga class should start with at least three minutes of meditation. Starting in mountain pose, everyone should close their eyes and place their hands in prayer position. Once everyone is in position, some gentle music can be added to enhance the experience.

Once this meditation is over, lead your class through several rounds of sun salutations. These can help loosen

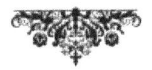

tight muscles and are a great way to reduce the risk of serious injuries as a class progresses.

Its important to make sure the entire body is adequately supple before starting any strength poses. While warrior poses are a pivotal part of a yoga practice, they can often cause strains in the legs if muscles aren't ready for them. Likewise, a raised leg downward dog can cause high levels of tension in the back and neck. By stretching these areas before going into an advanced pose, yoga teachers can reduce the risk of injuries to their students.

During the practice, it's important to make sure that each part of the body receives the same level of attention. If you're doing warrior poses or pigeon poses, it's essential to ensure that these exercises are completed on both sides of the body.

As the class progresses, you can increase the number of poses you do each minute. This provides a great cardiovascular workout for students. At the end of each session, students should remain in corpse pose for at least five minutes. This gives the body time to regenerate and allows students to reflect on the yoga session.

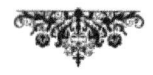

CHAPTER 5

TEACHING YOGA: CHALLENGES FOR KIDS IN YOGA

It is well known that Yoga is extremely beneficial for adults, but it can also be a great activity for children. Starting a Yoga practice, early in life, can give a child a head start on his or her health and well being. Some of the early benefits are conquering stress and obesity to set the foundation for a healthy adult life. However, Yoga can sometimes be seen as merely a 'grown-up' activity, so teaching it to children can come with some challenges.

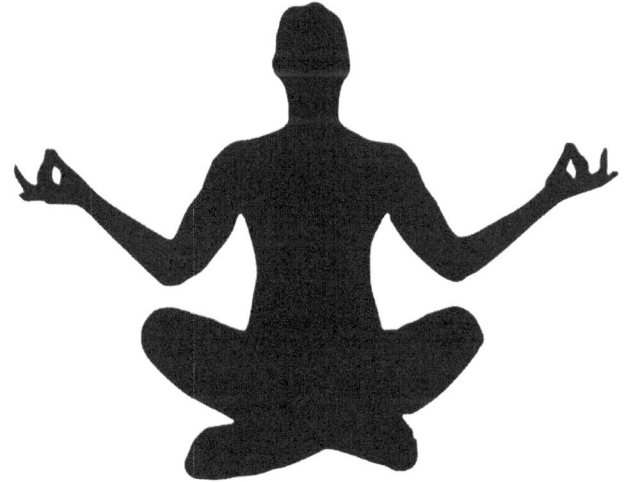

Teaching Yoga to Children

In order to properly practice Yoga, and receive the maximum benefits, the mind must be completely focused on the task at hand. The more concentration one applies to Yoga practice, the more benefits one will receive in the long run. Although, it is well known that children often have less than ideal attention spans, it is important for a teacher to capture their attention during a Yoga session. Keep the techniques brief and the meditation session short. Maintain the pace of the class by moving steadily from one technique to another. During meditation, it can also be useful to use a creative focus point, such as a stuffed animal or colorful picture on the wall.

When children are just starting out with Yoga practice, some of the techniques can seem very complicated to them. Always be sure to teach children proper breathing techniques so they can move through the poses with more ease. Start with introducing a few basic poses, such as Tree Pose or Child's Pose (how fitting!). Therefore, avoid overwhelming children by introducing too many new techniques in any given session.

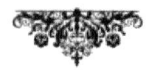

Precautions for a Safe Kids Yoga Class

Children can become anxious during their Yoga practice. While enthusiasm is very useful, it can also lead to injuries, in the form of joint injuries or strained muscles. Explain to children how to recognize their personal limitations and how to avoid pushing beyond their limits. To avoid strain, do not hold a pose for too long, and point out to the children that if they are feeling overexerted, to take a break.

The traditional quiet Yoga setting can spell boredom for some children. It is important to engage them in the physical exercise in order to reap the benefits, and for Yoga to become their cherished activity. Make up games and songs that teach Yoga principles. Practice some fast-paced Yoga (when a child is ready) to keep them challenged and engaged.

TEACHING YOGA FOR TEEN STRESS MANAGEMENT - FAMILY BONDS

Teens will respond to a Yoga class, with their peers, above all other age groups. Unless they have a nurturing personality, teens are not usually a good fit in a kids Yoga class. Sometimes, after-school activities, in high schools

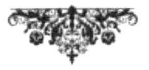

24

or junior high schools, will have Yoga as a choice. If there is no demand for teen Yoga classes in your area, adult classes will be the next best thing.

Over the years, it has been observed that concerned parents are puzzled by the sudden lack of communication with teens at home. This is usually a critical point in human life, as teens look over the horizon, toward adulthood. Suddenly, the "happy go lucky" attitude changes to a serious drone.

Many parents feel as if their teen has become a stranger. What can parents do to help their teens? One solution is to find joint activities, for parents and children, long before they become teens. This reinforces bonds during critical points in the lives of both parent and child.

Yoga is one such activity, but there are many more. Some families go hiking, skiing, biking, or participate in a variety of sports, together. There is no limit to the number of activities, but parent's should make a concerted effort to resist the role of a demanding coach. Turning a fun activity, into a pressure situation, is one sure way to force someone to drop out of it.

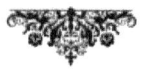

This is why Yoga is such a nice fit for the parent / child relationship. If you throw competition out the window, Yoga is an individual learning process. The rewards of a family practice are good health and re-establishing family ties.

COMPASSION FOR STUDENTS

You see it often: The child who cries, "No!" when someone attempts to squash a spider on the wall; the woman who tears up as she watches a mom hug her boy goodbye on the first day of kindergarten. Compassion (loving kindness) is a feeling that comes from within. Compassionate people can easily put themselves into the shoes of others, sympathizing with how they might feel in a variety of situations. When you feel compassion for others, you have a desire to help those in distress because you can imagine how you would feel in a similar situation. Some people are naturally more compassionate than others, but there are ways to cultivate those feelings within you to be a more effective Yoga teacher.

Showing compassion for others is an important part of creating a Yogic and non-threatening teaching

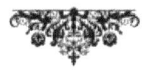

environment. Students can tell when the Yoga instructor truly cares about them and their well-being. Sometimes, students are disruptive, poor listeners, or just cannot seem to perform Yoga techniques correctly. In these situations, a compassionate Yoga teacher reaches out and helps with the utmost levels of kindness and patience. A non-compassionate teacher becomes annoyed, speaks sharply, or ignores those in need.

Yoga teachers can increase their level of compassion for others by practicing it on a regular basis. Practicing loving kindness is much like practicing a new Yoga posture. The more compassion you show toward others, the easier it becomes. Compassion can also be nurtured through your personal practice in daily life. There are a number of Yoga poses that are said to help bring compassion into your life. Heart opening, or back bending, asanas are said to increase our levels of compassion.

Pranayama techniques can also be extremely helpful for slowing the mind, clearing your thoughts, and allowing you to focus on showing more compassion to others. Pranayama can help bring inner peace and calm. Compassionate people often possess an inner calm that

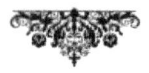

allows them to see beyond their own wants and needs to focus on others.

It is also important to show loving kindness toward yourself. Learn to avoid taking yourself too seriously. One of the hardest techniques to master is learning to laugh at one's self. Give yourself a break when you miscue a pose during class, fall out of a pose early, or mess up the sequence of poses. Students will understand that you are not perfect. When you show compassion toward yourself, you are able to laugh these little things off and press on.

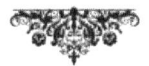

CHAPTER 6

GENERAL STUDENT SAFETY PRECAUTIONS

Y oga is considered healing for injuries, but that does not mean the potential for damage does not exist. Accidents and injuries are possible in every Yoga class, and instructors must be aware and take steps to minimize these problems. Beginner classes are especially fraught with potential for injury: Students unfamiliar with any particular movement have the potential to push themselves too far, fall from an unstable position, or try to compete with the practitioner on the next mat.

Here are some general student safety precautions for Yoga instructors:

Be aware, by watching your student's at all times. While teaching Yoga, the number one priority should be the safety of your students, rather than your own practice. Demonstrate the asana, and then come out of the position to observe the students. Move around the room, if all of the students are not visible to you. Consider the class level, and be especially vigilant with beginners and midlevel students. Keep class sizes small enough to feel comfortable watching everyone.

Recognize the potential for injuries. Some asanas lend themselves more to injuries, if not performed correctly. A pulled hamstring, for example, is a common injury in Yoga and is usually caused by overstretching in a seated or standing forward bend. Before moving into the posture, instruct student's to stretch slowly, not to jerk or bounce, and to stop at their comfort level.

Ask about pre-existing conditions, and design a questionnaire that addresses these questions, for the sake of student safety. Students may be relying on the Yoga teacher to tell them not to perform an asana with a pre-existing condition, but there should be a state of student and teacher awareness of the exact contraindication, when you warn them against the technique.

Prepare the muscles and joints for practice. Always complete a thorough warm-up before moving into the class. The length of the warm-up should be proportional to the skill level, with new student classes taking the longest. Age of the student, and time of day, are also factors in warming up. For example: Morning chair Yoga

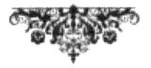

classes, with the median student, age of 75 years, require a longer warm-up than an evening beginner class, with a median student age of 25. This warm-up time not only prepares the body, it gives the mind time to focus, which is good for those new to Yoga. Setting intentions, and reminding students to listen to their bodies, can also help reduce injury rates.

THE IMPORTANCE OF TEACHING YOGA STUDENT SAFETY

Yoga is growing in popularity every single day as one of the best ways to get in great physical shape and rejuvenate the mind and body. However, due to the physical demands of yoga, it is important for every yoga instructor to emphasize yoga student safety in all yoga classes.

Many yoga newbies make the assumption that yoga is easy and not as physically demanding on the body as other forms of exercise. Just because yoga students are not constantly jumping around and running in place certainly does not demonstrate the intense physical nature of yoga and how serious injury is very possible.

Sprains, bone spurs and nerve damage are just a few examples of how students can become injured when they

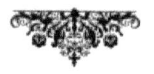

do not practice yoga properly. While more severe injuries are not commonplace, they do happen. Luckily, there are some very easy steps that instructors can take to ensure safety in their classes.

The first thing an instructor must do is properly teach each yoga pose. In addition to simply demonstrating how to perform the exercise, instructors should always teach the proper way for the body to move and how far it should extend to prevent injury. Instructors should also teach warning signs of possible injury. Some students may not realize the difference in pain that comes from working hard and pain from pushing the body too hard.

It is a common practice for yoga instructors to personally assist their students with yoga poses. This is something that every yoga instructor should do to make sure students are performing poses as they should. This will help students to understand what position their body should be in when performing the pose. Obviously, yoga instructors cannot feel the pain that may be occurring with students during yoga poses and should never push students too hard. Yoga safety really begins with those who teach the instructors.

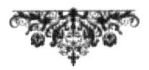

Another important aspect of teaching yoga safety with students is for the instructor to be familiar with their student's medical history. If students have existing injuries, certain yoga poses may cause further injury. If the class size is small enough, the instructor can more easily keep track of any history of injury with their student's and can advise proper yoga poses throughout the class for individual students. In larger classes, the instructor should be aware of each pose and how it could aggravate injury. For example, if a certain yoga pose may be difficult for someone with a back injury, the yoga instructor should advise students as a group of such potential for injury.

Instructors should always be mindful of the fact that there will be students in their classes who are over-achievers. These students may push themselves a little harder than they should. Good instructors should closely watch all their students and intervene when they feel as though a student is pushing themselves beyond their limits.

Yoga student safety should be the first concern for every yoga instructor before each class begins. A well-educated

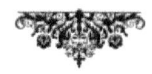

instructor who has their student's best interest at heart will ensure a successful and safe yoga experience for everyone.

CHAPTER 7

TEACHING YOGA TO PREGNANT STUDENTS

Pregnant students should be in a specialized class with a teacher who has successfully completed a prenatal yoga teacher training course. This is the reason why so many yoga classes begin with health warnings concerning pregnancy. You have the right to refuse to teach any person who is putting their health at risk.

Yoga is a great way for pregnant women to stay active, limber and calm. Women experiencing a healthy pregnancy can feasibly do yoga right up to the delivery date. Some expecting moms even find comfort in yoga poses and meditation during labor. It's always important for women to check in with their doctors first to ensure that yoga training is a safe choice for them. Beyond that, there are a few other precautions to take as the pregnancy progresses. Prenatal yoga instructors must be highly aware of the cautions and teach their mommies accordingly.

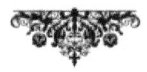

The First Trimester

During the first trimester of pregnancy, a woman's body is undergoing massive amounts of change. Hormones are shifting to accommodate the growing fetus. Common side effects include nausea, fatigue and tenderness around the breasts. Most of these changes occur within the body, leaving a woman's appearance greatly unchanged. Most women can engage in yoga exactly as they did before they were pregnant. Pregnant women should make sure to drink plenty of water and to pay attention to their bodies for any discomfort. They should never push their selves beyond their limits during pregnancy. The top precaution would be to avoid jumping

The Second Trimester

The second trimester typically brings a sense of normalcy and peace as women's bodies have finally adjusted to pregnancy. Although the belly begins to protrude, most women have gotten over the feelings of nausea and tenderness associated with the early weeks of pregnancy. There are a few more precautions for yoga practice during this trimester.

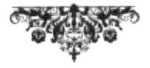

As the body prepares for the upcoming birth, women's joints and ligaments tend to become ultra lubricated. This can be a concern because women might get into a situation where they are putting their selves at risk of injury for pushing too far into a stretch. Women should proceed into each pose slowly and with caution. Movements should be slow and calculated. They should also avoid any poses that require lying flat on their backs to ensure adequate blood flow to the uterus at all times.

The Third Trimester

The last weeks of pregnancy can become uncomfortable for women as their bellies become unbearably large. A woman's balance will most likely be a little of during the third trimester. She should go into balance poses carefully, with the aide of a wall or chair nearby. Props might also be useful to help accommodate the protruding belly and maintain poses comfortably. Pregnant women should remember to keep moving during the routine and not hold any one pose for too long. Again, women should avoid lying flat on their backs, choosing a side-lying position instead. It's also important to avoid lying on the stomach.

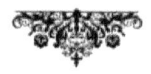

THE DRAMA OF A YOGA SCHOOL AS A BUSINESS

So, you want to open a yoga school? The popularity of yoga is a huge incentive for people of all walks of life to become a yoga teacher, teach as an independent contractor, start a yoga school, or leave their day jobs behind. However, what looks easy to many people needs some planning. Businesses open and close in a few months because of bad locations, no business plan, there are not enough funds to sustain a start up, marketing budgets, and many more possibilities.

Obtaining Certification

According to industry standard, the first step on your journey to launching your own yoga school should be to obtain certification as an instructor from an accredited institution. Becoming certified usually means that you are in for a big education. For years, nobody was certified until yoga instructors realized that they could be sued. That's right - in some countries, suing is like the lottery. Today is your lucky day, because you can sue anybody for anything. Lawyers love it, while some people diligently plan and scheme for their opportunity to take anybody to court.

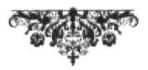

38

What can yoga instructors do? Get certified, get covered by a liability insurance company, and establish a track record of safe procedures in your classes. Registration is an option, but its not often required for liability insurance. To be honest, some teachers (who are not certified or registered) have sports liability insurance coverage. However, certification does show that you are formally educated in safely teaching yoga classes. So, that does build your credibility as a yoga teacher who cares about student safety.

Create A Plan Of Action

Once you are certified, research the fees charged for yoga instruction in your demographic, to stay competitive and create a plan of action! In addition, you must decide if you would like to be the sole proprietor of your yoga school, be a partner, incorporate or run a limited liability company. It is essential to work out the details of this part of the business since new instructors income may vary from $30,000 to $70,000 a year. As a sole proprietor, you can build a private clientele to gain exposure and build rapport that may actually prove more lucrative.

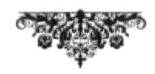

There is also the option to be an independent contractor. As an independent contractor you can work as a sole proprietor from an existing building, such as a private health club, or fitness center, with a built-in clientele, to avoid the overhead costs associated with renting your own building and paying for staff. You will also need to determine what type of yoga you will teach at your school and specialize in that. In a health club, people want to achieve different things through yoga and may not choose to participate in yogic breathing or meditation, but may prefer the physical flexibility and strength training aspect of this discipline instead. Popular yoga workouts for fitness centers include Vinyasa, Hot Yoga, Ashtanga and Power Yoga.

Where's the Drama?

Regardless of the path a yoga business takes, there are some key factors to be mindful of: Seek the credentials and licenses needed to get started, choose a plan of marketing, the type of yoga that will best suit your clients, and carefully advertise your business based on your chosen discipline. In addition, purchase insurance that covers the type of yoga school you are running, to protect yourself legally.

True to ancient yogic philosophy, it takes a lot of dedication and hard work to make any business a reality. Beyond the poses, meditation, spiritual enlightenment, mantras, and breathing exercises, yoga has become increasingly trendy, and is now an industry, according to the New York Times. The drama is the daily management of time, energy, personalities, and money. If you think becoming a yoga teacher has nothing to do with business, you will be in for a big surprise.

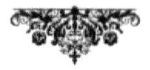

CHAPTER 8

YOGA TEACHERS CAN PREVENT INJURIES

Most Yoga teachers are certified instructors, who have gone through a lengthy training process, in order to be qualified to teach Yoga. If you have not already done so, you should look into Yoga teacher training courses to undergo the proper training to support your status as instructor. Typically, an advanced Yoga practitioner, who has years of experience, needs intensive training before being qualified to teach. However, even qualified Yoga instructors might be in need of strategies to help reduce, or prevent, injuries in their classrooms.

When Yoga Injuries Occur

Practitioners are most at risk for injury - when attempting a Yoga pose too challenging for their strength or health level, when doing a pose incorrectly, when not warmed up, or when distracted or unable to focus. As a result, Yoga teachers must remember that their primary job as instructors is not to perfect their own Yoga practice, but to keep their students focused, while they practice a variety of Yogic techniques safely.

Yoga Class Sizes

The size of of the class can impact an instructor's ability to teach Yoga effectively. For example: If a beginner Yoga class is too big, the instructor may be unable to give enough attention to each student, as needed. As a result - beginner and youth classes should be smaller, with intermediate and advanced classes, allowing more Yoga students per session to balance business needs. Similarly, participation in athletic schools of Yoga makes injuries more likely, so teachers in these schools will see fewer injuries in classes that have smaller student-to-instructor ratios.

Feedback

To prevent injuries from occurring, instructors need to be completely focused on teaching, especially paying attention to each student's technique and alignment. Good correction tends to be in-depth and verbal, rather than physical, since students might lose their balance if you make the change for them or may be uncomfortable with physical correction.

What to Watch For

Yoga instructors should be on the lookout for certain behaviors to help prevent student injuries.

First - since Yoga injuries happen when students are distracted, teachers should be careful to guide their students in concentration techniques to encourage focus. Instructors should not hesitate to speak with a distracted student if the issue does not resolve quickly.

Second - since injuries also happen when Yoga practitioners push themselves beyond what they can handle, teachers should take care to emphasize a slow mastery of poses, and to demonstrate this themselves, with the free use of props. Some practitioners feel embarrassed using props or get frustrated, if they do not move on to more complicated poses quickly; therefore, Yoga instructors must take care to model the safest practice techniques themselves.

Third - instructors should watch for trembling or wobbling, especially in balancing poses, since this can indicate muscle fatigue or weakness. Encouraging students who are tired, or too fatigued, to rest will help

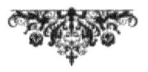

them avoid injuries that result from incorrect Yoga techniques, improper alignment, or falling.

WHAT ARE THE BENEFITS OF A YIN YOGA TEACHER COURSE?

Many yoga enthusiasts, even those who have refined their practice and made it a part of their daily lives, never seriously consider enrolling in a teacher training course. Since most people begin a serious yoga practice with the intent of bettering themselves instead of seeking a new career, many candidates who would be perfect for a teacher training program like the Yin yoga teacher course never even seek out more information about this wonderful opportunity.

Just because you aren't ready to give up your current job and devote your entire life to yoga doesn't mean that you aren't necessarily a candidate for training to teach it. In fact, many yogis seek out this training, even if they aren't considering teaching as their main profession. Here are some benefits of enrolling in a yoga teacher training program.

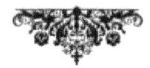

Take Your Practice To New Heights - Teacher training certainly involves learning about how to be a good instructor. Beyond that, however, it will help experienced yogis to take their practice to a whole new level. Future teachers learn advanced poses and techniques to help novices perfect their practice. The best way to learn is by teaching. Because of this, many yogis find that they are able to perform new poses and improve their current practice thanks to a teacher training program, even if they never go on to actually instruct in a class setting.

Don't Have To Give Up Your Career - Just because you undergo training doesn't mean that you have to give up your current career. There are many licensed yoga instructors who keep their regular job, obtaining the training merely for the sake of perfecting their yoga practice. With teacher training under your belt, you will also have the option to consider instructing yogis part-time. There are plenty of yoga instructors who just give part-time instruction or one-on-one sessions while still working their regular job.

Obtain a New Outlook on Your Practice - Nothing compares to a training course when it comes to really changing your outlook on your entire yoga practice.

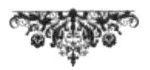

Teacher training helps students to really understand the benefits of yoga, from the physical to the spiritual. You'll meet advanced instructors who truly understand the mind-body connection of yoga. The entire experience will help you to see your yoga practice with a new level of enlightenment.

If you are preparing to begin your Yin yoga teacher training program, begin the process with an open mind. Even if you are a very experienced yoga practitioner, approaching yoga from a teaching perspective is a whole other animal. A yoga practitioner approaches yoga with the mindset of bettering his or herself, while an instructor approaches their practice with the outlook of guiding a group of people along their yoga journey. This group approach, however, is a great way for any yogi to approach class instruction. Connecting with others on your personal yoga journey can be one of the most meaningful aspects of your practice.

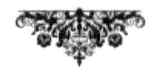

CHAPTER 9

WHAT ARE THE ADVANTAGES OF BECOMING A YOGA TEACHER?

Yoga is the art and technology of treatment and as more people discover the several health and fitness advantages of yoga, there prevails a constant need for certified yoga instructors. If you have obtained the wonderful real, psychological and spiritual health and fitness advantages of yoga for yourself, you may choose to become an instructor to help others do the same.

Yoga as an alternative treatment exercise has benefits, both for the yoga instructor and the student. However, in order to obtain these benefits, yoga needs to be applied consistently under the management of a yoga instructor, making this an ideal profession option.

What are the Advantages of becoming a Yoga Teacher?

A natural result of becoming a yoga instructor is that it will help you take your yoga exercise to a whole new stage

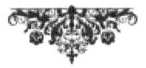

with innovative methods and poses that will improve your own health and fitness.

It is known that the right way to learn is to educate others and by using your recently obtained abilities, you can help beginners obtain perfection in their individual yoga methods to heal their bodies of accidents and other conditions.

Teaching yoga will considerably improve your power and make you fit and strong.

The multi-size things of the exercise of yoga will provide your personal satisfaction as your learners experience health improvements that boost their power and make them feel fit and strong.

As a yoga instructor, you will become a living testimony through which the many benefits of yoga can be seen by those looking for real, psychological and spiritual well-being.

As a yoga instructor, you will not be confined to exercising in a particular place as it can be performed

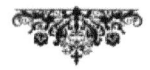

world-wide and you can take your profession with you wherever you go.

Yoga's meditation element is best for soothing the thoughts, obtaining serenity, resolving emotional stress and connecting to the inner spirit. Sharing these meditation benefits with others will provide you a feeling of serenity in the knowledge that you are assisting people on a worldwide level.

The financial benefits of becoming a yoga instructor can be quite important as there is a requirement for competent instructors.

As a yoga instructor, you will be able to exercise and improve on your problem solving abilities as well as organizational abilities as you endeavor to become a better instructor.

As a yoga instructor, you will be forced to keep your own thoughts and body in a sound condition and lead a well-organized way of life in order to pass the same to your learners.

Yoga will increase its impact well beyond the above benefits as it will impact your whole way of life, such as

your eating routines. In order to truly expert yoga, you will need to accept and follow the rules of yoga such as the yoga diet. Yogi diet plans are mostly veggie and some, but the main focus is on consuming food that is impressive, which benefits not only your body but the whole environment as well.

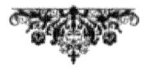

CHAPTER 10

TIPS ON HOW TO TEACH YOGA STUDENTS

Over the past decade, yoga has exploded in popularity. Some people use yoga as a way to stay in shape. Others use it as a method for relaxing and relieving stress. No matter where you live, there is a good chance there is a yoga class going on nearby. If you are a yoga instructor, there are many ways to go about passing on your knowledge to the people in your class. Let's take a look at some tips that deal with how to teach yoga students:

1. Arrive in your class early

Try to show up in each of your classes at least 15 minutes early. This will give your students time to ask you any questions they have about the previous class. They can also ask for your advice on any problems they are having in the class. This type of communication between the yoga student and the teacher will help the student get the most out of the class.

2. Focus on one topic per class

Some yoga instructors have a method of teaching where they like to jump around from one topic to another. They believe this helps the class flow better while not becoming boring or stale. However, these instructors are not thinking about the people who are slow learners or those individuals who are not in good shape. These people may take longer to learn a specific technique. Therefore, more time should be spent with them before moving on to the next posture or exercise. If someone is in a yoga class, there is a good chance that person has little or no knowledge of the various positions and movements. As an instructor, if you try to cram too many topics into one class, you are cheating your students and failing to teach them anything. Choose one topic and build the entire class around it. Only move on to a secondary topic if you are certain the entire class has mastered the first one.

3. Do not use medical terms for the anatomy

When you are a teacher, the most important thing is that all of your students understand you. If your students do not understand some of the terminologies you are using, they will not be getting the full benefit of your knowledge. It will also slow down your class if students are constantly asking what certain terms mean. Remember, this is a yoga

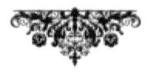

class, not a medical class. Therefore, make sure you use simple terms such as lower back, upper back, ribs, head, chest and stomach. Then you can be certain that all of your students will always know exactly what you mean.

4. Walk around the room as you teach

Many yoga instructors make the mistake of staying on their mat in front of the class while teaching. Walking around the room is more effective. This is especially important if you are teaching a large class with at least 50 people. As you walk around the room, take a close look at what each of your students is doing. Check to see if they are performing the postures or exercises correctly. If they are having difficulty, show them the right way to do it. You will not be able to see how the students, especially those located on the sides or at the back are doing unless you make the effort to closely inspect the entire class.

HOW TO TEACH YOGA STUDENTS WITH CONFIDENCE AND PATIENCE

Once you've finished your training to become a yoga instructor, you may be asking yourself "what do I do next?" You may have all the skills and knowledge, but you're about to teach a group of students for the first time.

Here are several ways on how to teach yoga students the right way and with confidence.

First, make sure to stop and take a breath. Students can tell when you're nervous as it shows in how you conduct business. The best way to calm your nerves is taking the time to relax. Calm yourself and take a breath before starting. Realize that public speaking rarely comes easy to anyone, but it will with practice. You will get used to it and it will be easier down the road.

When you're first getting your feet wet, the best way to plan your first classes is to keep it simple. The more complicated classes should come from having plenty of experience under your belt, as students would expect. I don't think anyone would enjoy taking an advanced course only to find out their teacher hasn't been teaching that long at all. It will be much easier to get the hang of things by starting simple and working your way up.

Go slow. If you're started afresh, the odds are the majority of your students are as well. You may have a few who already know the right posture and aren't intimidated by their first few times on the mat. Students new to yoga are

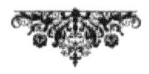

much like children who are starting their first year of school. Excited, but not sure what to expect. They may fall, get frustrated, but those sorts of things are easier to correct and ensure a repeat student if you are slow and show patience.

Stick to one theme. Jumping around from theme to theme will be difficult for you to keep track of and will be even harder for your students. Start a class revolving around one specific class and let that be your specialty. Also, keep to using familiar body names and terms, keeping it simple and easy to understand. Telling people about ardha chandrasana, people will become very confused.

Ask your students questions about their experience. There is no better way to learn how to teach yoga students than by making sure they had a pleasant experience. If you were confusing or something was too difficult, you can better adapt the way you do things. Open the floor by asking the class as a whole if they have any questions. By doing this, you show you actually care for the students and teaching them the right way that works for them. Also, it is how they will best learn the moves and become more experienced.

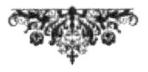

CHAPTER 11

HOW TO TEACH YOGA OR DEEPEN YOUR OWN
PRACTICE

I f you've been practicing yoga for some time now, you may have become interested in teaching yoga to other people, or in deepening your own yoga practice. But, as you may have learned, teaching yoga to others, or developing your own yoga practice, takes a different set of skills than those of a yoga student.

So, what makes a good yoga teacher? When students feel better about themselves after class than before class, you can feel good about what you are doing with them. On top of that, if you can help your students become more aware of their own bodies and emotions and more accepting of their body and emotions, you've done your job. Besides being a skillful teacher, a great yoga teacher is also an interested yoga student. It's important to establish and maintain your own daily practice to become a better teacher. There are certain things that you can never learn from books or from teaching others, that you can only learn (and pass onto your students) from consistently doing your own yoga practice.

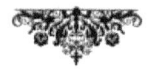

No matter what style of yoga you teach, you can follow certain guidelines to create a wonderful practice for your students or for yourself. By incorporating some of the following teaching strategies, you will improve the overall experience for your student's and yourself.

Set objectives and themes. Find out the needs of your class by asking students what they are looking to gain from yoga practice. This will help you determine if its more important to focus on certain themes, such as stress relieve, improving energy levels, back pain, strength, flexibility, etc. Set themes for your own practice, so you have a different focus each time and keep it interesting.

Learn and share the benefits of specific yoga postures and breathing exercises. Studies have shown that educating student's about their bodies and the effects of the exercises they are doing increases motivation and exercise compliance. Learning about specific benefits will increase your motivation too.

Remind students (and yourself) to breath and to focus on their breath throughout their practice. When holding a

difficult pose, we all have a tendency to hold our breath. Remind your students (or yourself) to breathe fully and deeply. Focusing on the breath also brings attention inward and can deepen a practice by stilling the mind and putting you more in touch with the present moment.

Practice effective presentation skills. Okay, this one is just for those who are planning to teach others. Remember to make eye contact with individual students throughout the class. Be sure to make eye contact with all parts of the classroom. Stand tall with your arms relaxed at your sides to convey confidence, yet openness.

Know your material. The only way to truly feel confident teaching yoga or to develop your own practice is to know your material. This means understanding the effects of the yoga poses and breathing exercises you teach and practice, and understanding how their benefits, as well as understanding the philosophy and history behind yoga.

HOW TO TEACH YOGA IN THE CORPORATE MARKETPLACE

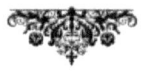

For most Yoga teachers, bragging does not come easy. Yet, the public cannot see the obvious benefits of Yoga, unless you point them out. When you decided to become a Yoga teacher, you also decided to educate the public about Yoga.

When Yoga instructors mention these points in their marketing materials, this becomes an offer that defines Yoga's many benefits, instead of supposing that a corporate decision maker knows what Yoga is. When it comes down to it, you should be able to explain the benefits of Yoga in a paragraph and have it etched into your memory.

This prepares you when you talk to the public about what you do. To state: "I teach Yoga classes," is not enough of an explanation - if the person you talk to has a mental picture of Yoga as just a bunch of pretzel poses, displayed by show-offs.

Your letters, to local companies, should be as long as needed, but you should also mention the benefits of having a corporate Yoga program in the first paragraph or two. The decision maker, who reads your letter, will see

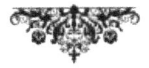

the benefits, or not, but if you have captured his or her interest, he or she will continue to read.

You could refer potential companies to your Yoga website, as well. However, if you have captured a prospective decision maker's attention, you had better fully explain the benefits of a Corporate Yoga program, while you have captured his or her attention.

I can already hear the complaints, "I wanted to become a Yoga teacher, not a copywriter." If you can talk, you can write. After you write, have your copy proof read, a few times, by someone who is good at it. If you really need a copywriter, feel free to contact me, but please understand that quality copywriting is not cheap.

Let's get back to the types of injuries Yoga workshops can prevent. For office workers, Yoga can help stretch out connective tissues in the wrists, hands, fingers, elbows, shoulders, neck, and back. All of these areas can stiffen up through repetitive motion. Add to this fact, that all of an office worker's muscle groups can become very tense and create backaches, headaches, anxiety, hyper tension, and many more ailments.

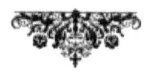

Manufacturing companies, with workers who assemble products, also see a multitude of injuries - from industrial accidents to repetitive motion injuries - specific to the job. Yoga instructors can teach how to shift weight properly without injury. Developing awareness, or "living in the moment," can also help reduce accidents.

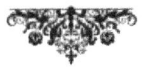

CHAPTER 12

WHY IS TEACHING YOGA SO REWARDING?

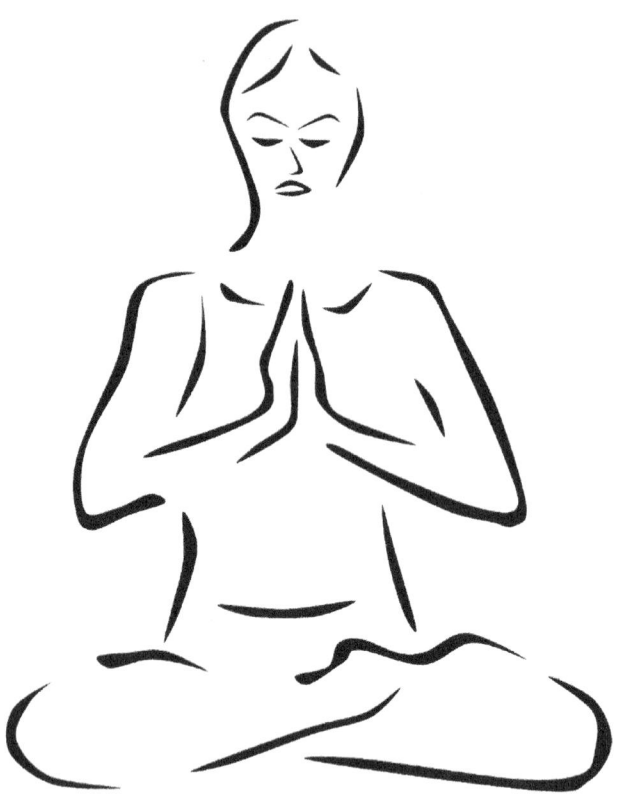

Can teaching Yoga really be that rewarding? Why do Yoga teachers love their job? Will your Yoga training open up doors for your dream job? Let's look at some of these questions and see how you can make your dream job become a reality. Even if you have no desire to teach Yoga, the practice of Yoga can be your gateway to satisfaction, fulfillment, achievement, and a successful life.

Is teaching Yoga classes really a rewarding occupation? After the first student comes up and thanks you for class - that is only the beginning. Some Yoga students have pre-existing ailments and pain. Yoga cannot promise a cure for any ailment, but Yoga can offer less pain, pain management, and sometimes, pain goes away altogether. Your students will definitely tell you what Yoga does for them.

The gratification of helping others, on a daily basis, is spontaneous. This cultivates positive energy from within the core of your inner being. You give the gift of Yoga, but you share positive energy, and usually walk away with more energy than you had before you taught a Yoga class.

Being able to make your own hours is a priceless benefit for Yoga teachers. You do not have to be in traffic during peak times. You choose the time and place you want to work. If you want to teach Yoga in the morning at a corporate fitness center, senior center, health club, or teach a private Yoga session, you can choose the best option for your schedule and "pocket book."

As a Yoga teacher, you are a perennial student for life. You must pursue knowledge every day, for the safety of your students, to enhance your Yoga teaching practice, and to improve the lives of all those who learn from you. TIPS ON HOW TO TEACH YOGA STUDENTS ON THE FIRST DAY

There are many resources available that suggest how to teach yoga students. But if students don't return for the second day, it's all a waste of time. An instructor has just a couple of hours to convince their students that this will be a life-changing experience and that they are the person that can guide them there. Understanding this keeps classes full of curious and dedicated students.

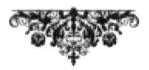

Make a Connection

An instructor that can express how yoga has improved their life gets students interested. It doesn't need to be a story of cancer survival. It could be that yoga helps concentration while in college. Perhaps it calmed anxieties around relationships. Or it even could have been a way to better health. A connection is made with the instructor when the students hear that yoga has the potential of helping them in their everyday lives.

Less Talk and More Doing

The classroom contains a variety of students. Different physical attributes, backgrounds, cultures and experience levels are present. Each student has different questions that will take the entire session to answer. They all share one thing - they are there to do yoga. After a short introduction, show them a breath or warm up technique and "hit the mats."

Target the Beginners

When the class has multiple levels of experience, focus on the beginners. The experienced students know the limits of their bodies. They know how to match their breath with the pose. Help the beginning student master the basics. It

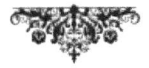

will motivate others in the class to perfect their techniques.

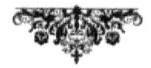

Everyone Will Be Successful

When an instructor looks at the class with this thought, they work with the strength of each student. One student may be quick to pick up on a breath exercise. Another may adopt the Mountain pose perfectly the first time. Some students will succeed just by having tried all the exercises and made it to the end of the class. When each student feels that they have had a successful yoga session, they will be back.

Give Them Something to Take From the Class

Students with little motivation to think about yoga after the first class may not be back for the next one. Give them a simple Pranayama exercise such as abdominal breath or alternative nostril breath to do at home. Show them Child's pose and have them do this every morning. Give them something to remind them of yoga each day before the next class. They will be back to see what else they can take away and use in their lives.

Perfection Comes from Practice

However well the students follow the exercises on the first day is perfect for them in that session. Don't be concerned about perfect arm and leg positions. Don't

suggest that yoga is not really being done properly until they do attain perfect control of their bodies. Encourage the students to practice. Praise them for having a successful first class. Every student wants to hear "You did great today and you'll do even better in the next class."

Be the Student

Learning how to teach yoga students is something an instructor continues doing throughout their career. Each student provides different challenges. Each student learns differently. The instructor who recognizes this is flexible, adaptable and always asking themselves how they can improve their teaching skills.

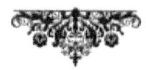

CHAPTER 13

THE PERSEVERANCE OF TEACHING YOGA

Why do talented students fall short of becoming Yoga teachers? Ever notice that "quick flashes" of brilliance disappear in a short time. Take for example, the super flexible Yoga student who can do a split in every direction, and make a pretzel, or circle, out of his, or her, body on the first Yoga class. Usually, this student will leave after the first class saying, "Is that all there is to Yoga?"

As most of us know there is so much more to Yoga than mere flexibility, but how do you make a student aware of this in his or her first Yoga class? Do you really want to try? Some Yoga teachers jump through "flaming hoops" to appease a potential student who has natural flexibility. This happens much to the dismay of dedicated and established Yoga students who have been training for years.

So what is the problem and why do we worship exceptional flexibility and physical prowess? The problem stems from the Yoga teacher who has forgotten

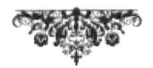

what the prime ingredient is within the exceptional Yoga student. That ingredient is "perseverance" and that is what separates the "flash in the pan" from the Yoga student who may well evolve into a Yoga teacher. The student who shows up to Yoga class and tries to do his, or her, best should never be taken for granted.

Perseverance is a true guarantee of success for Yoga students and Yoga teachers alike. When you think about your life, perseverance has always played a major role in your past achievements. How many people will tell you that teaching Yoga is not a good career move? Plenty will, but you must have the fortitude and perseverance to pursue your own desire, in the first place.

In order to make any achievement in Yoga, you need a formula for success. Here is a list of ingredients that you must have in order to succeed at teaching Yoga or anything else in life. Firstly, you need desire and passion to become a Yoga teacher. If you don't have it, that's no problem, just find something that you feel passionate about. Do not waste time pursuing any goal without passion.

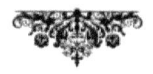

Secondly you must have a dream that you can visualize. If you can picture yourself teaching Yoga, and feel the joy of your journey, you are fine. However, if you cannot see yourself becoming a Yoga teacher, it just might not be your "calling." Whatever the goals you choose to pursue in life, you will need both desire and the ability to visualize your dreams, in order to proceed to the next step.

HOW MUCH DO YOGA INSTRUCTORS GET PAID?

Within Yoga teacher circles, most instructors never discuss their annual income. Salaries can be a "touchy subject;" particularly when one has a vocation in the arts or embracing the spiritual aspects of Yoga. All of these are viewed as enjoyable "hobbies," but can have a professional aspect. Many imagine that they would love to get paid to teach Yoga, and some of us have this reality. Yet, what kind of salary expectation is reasonable, and how can a Yoga teacher support a family in an uncertain economy?

According to payscale.com, hourly wages for Yoga teacher's range from $10.33 to $54.25 an hour. If we do the math, this leads one to think an annual salary of

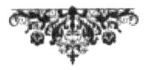

between $23,000 - $113,000 is about right. This range, however, is wide enough to render the statistics meaningless. On the lower end, the salary is approximately poverty level for a family of four. On the upper end, it is an extraordinary salary, on which living comfortably would be very easy. To make sense of the numbers, it is necessary to delve deeper.

The High End of Teaching Yoga

First, the overall job market for Yoga instructors should be considered. If you are at the lower end of the pay scale, it is not worth much to know that someone is paid over $100 an hour, but those jobs are rare. Bikram lives well, but his students are often actresses, actors, and professionals. Some Yoga teacher's work with professional athletes and executives in Fortune 500 companies. To know that these positions exist is not enough. Reaching out to students or clients, who pay handsomely for your services, is a marketing strategy that most Yoga teachers do not want to indulge in.

The Internal Conflict of Getting Paid

To some teachers, taking any payment is awkward and might be viewed as greedy or wrong. Students, who want

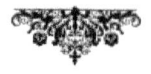

free Yoga sessions, often take the position of refusing to compensate one's teacher. Some people sincerely feel that all Yoga teachers should live an ascetic or monastic lifestyle and take a vow of poverty. As Yoga continues to expand in popularity, many contemporary forms exist, and most modern instructors have not taken a vow of poverty. Anecdotally, it is well known that most Yoga instructors are paid hourly, rather than by salary. Most Yoga instructors, who have discussed their salaries in personal blogs or magazine articles, offer a standard income of $29,000- $35,000 annually.

Common earning scenarios, for teaching Yoga classes, include five different options - although there are many more.

1) The Yoga teacher pays a rental fee to the studio, and keeps any fees paid by students, who pay the teacher directly.

2) The teacher is paid a portion of the class fees, which are typically 50-75%, and the students pay the studio.

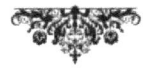

3) The Yoga instructor is paid a flat fee for teaching, by the studio, regardless of the number of students.

4) A combination of the above - often a flat fee plus a premium for every student beyond a certain threshold.

5) Private, individual classes taught outside a studio, to an individual student, for which the student pays the Yoga teacher directly.

Private classes can be considered the most effective for students, and the most lucrative for teachers, but are by their nature limited in quantity. Other earning opportunities depend on the teaching scenario and the market for Yoga in the teacher's geographic area.

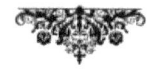

CHAPTER 14

TEACHING YOGA AND ACCEPTING CHANGE

T eaching your Yoga students to accept changes, throughout life, may be their most difficult task to put into practice. Luckily, Yoga is designed to help people cope with new situations, which occur on a daily basis. The practice of Yoga is a great tool for helping a practitioner to accept change.

Often, we are so busy that we are not even aware of the changes that are occurring within us and around us. Yoga helps us to slow our body, breath and mind down, so that we can become aware of our own physical and emotional state. Our bodies change daily, even hourly, sometimes we have a tremendous amount of energy and on other days, we are very tired or fatigued and need a more restorative practice.

The art of the practice of Yoga is based on the self-awareness of what we actually need in the moment. The practice of ahimsa, or non-violence is a core element of Yoga. Once you become aware of what you need, the key is to choose a sequence of asanas, pranayama, and

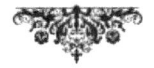

meditation that truly nourish you and are appropriate for you on a given day. In order to be aware of the changing nature of our present needs, we must learn to tune into our emotional and physical state of being without judgment. This includes a compassionate awareness of the changing state of our bodies and minds on a daily basis.

For example, to work in a kitchen preparing meals for two hundred retreat participant's at a Yoga conference, and then engage in a vigorous two hour Yoga practice, may not be appropriate or even self-loving. You may need a much more restorative practice after a long day in the kitchen. In this context, the concept of success is self-referential. In other words, a successful practice is based on an evaluation of how well you match the practice you create to what your body, mind and spirit may need on any given day.

There are also times in our lives when we are recovering from an illness, injury or surgical procedure when we need to engage in a much more gentle Yoga practice than we are used to doing. These limitations can be very frustrating and difficult to accept, especially if you are used to engaging in a vigorous practice of Yoga. As we

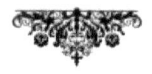

go through the decades of our lives, the needs of our bodies and minds also change and evolve.

As we decide to pass the torch to others, teaching Yoga helps us to accept change, because the practice itself makes us slow down enough to become aware of the changes that have occurred and supports us in tailoring our teaching and practice to our current physical, while calming our emotional state. We are constantly reminded to breathe deeply, look within, and find out what is true for us in that moment. To move through life from that inner place of ahimsa is what each of us is taught at our foundational Yoga teacher training.

TEACHING YOGA AND FINDING A MENTOR

One of the ways that Yoga teachers grow, and learn, in their profession is by finding a mentor. A mentor teacher is usually someone with a few more years of experience; someone who excels at what they do; and someone wishing to enrich the teaching skills of a younger Yoga instructor.

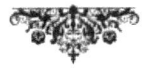

Teaching Yoga requires a complex set of skills, knowledge, and methods that are best learned through practice. The best Yoga teachers improve, and progress, as they gain experience in the studio or ashram. A mentor teacher can provide valuable advice and knowledge to less experienced instructors, and a place for the new Yoga teacher to voice frustrations and concerns.

Find a mentor that you admire. Usually, you can spot mentor-worthy Yoga teachers by the way they run their class, the way their students feel about them, or by the way they make you feel when interacting with them. Approach a potential mentor by letting them know how you admire their teaching methods, and how you aspire to be able to teach in a manner that is similar to theirs. Ask if they would be interested in mentoring you, as you begin your journey as a Yoga instructor.

You might begin by asking to observe their class. Focus your observation on one thing at a time. One class you might hone-in on is how your mentor interacts with students, and during another, you might consider the cues given for each pose. Take notes as you observe, noting methods or comments you liked, and any questions you

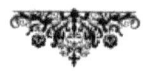

have for your mentor. Spend time after class discussing ideas. Have an open mind, and try to absorb all the advice you can. Although you won't use all the ideas your mentor gives you, eventually, you will assimilate all of these skills with your own Yoga practice.

You can also ask your mentor to watch you, in action, while teaching. Ask him or her to note anything that didn't quite work, or any concerns they see in your practice. Be willing to take criticism and advice - knowing that it will help you become a better teacher in the long run.

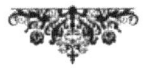

CHAPTER 15

TEACH YOGA STUDENTS TO MANAGE BACK PAIN

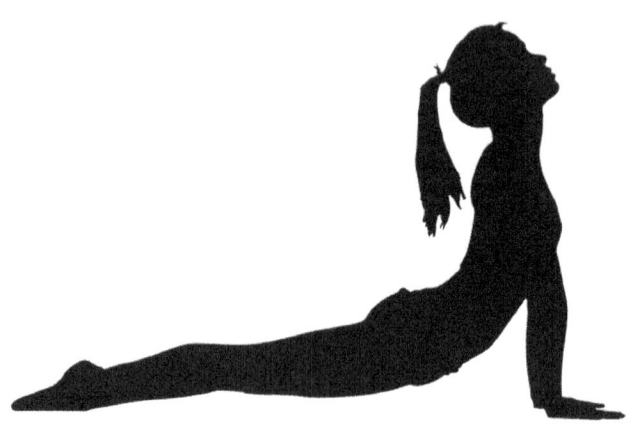

When you teach yoga classes, how often do students ask about techniques to reduce back pain? Study after study shows that yoga helps significantly with managing back pain in conjunction with medical treatment. Yoga strengthens and balances the body while it grants students more control of their minds. Each of these factors alone become huge benefits, when dealing with back pain, but together, they feel like a miracle. Participants of one study reported a decrease in pain, functional disability, and depression. Sixty-eight percent of the participant's of that study assigned to practice yoga also continued to practice the art after the study concluded. Even though chronic back pain can be one of the hardest common conditions to live with and treat, yoga can significantly improve the quality of life of back pain sufferers.

One form of yoga commonly practiced to deal with back pain is Restorative yoga; it has specifically been shown to improve mood as well as lessen the pain. Restorative is a therapeutic form of yoga. It strengthens muscles and brings the body into alignment. It is exercise, and like any exercise, it releases dopamine, which vastly improves the mood of the person exercising. This effect is so strong that exercise has been found in scientific studies to be a more effective treatment for depression than drugs in all but the most extreme cases. It is the ultimate mood-booster and promoter of well-being.

Restorative is a contemporary form of yoga specifically developed for therapeutic purposes and many studies have reported excellent results with its use. Viniyoga and Iyengar yoga, are also used to treat back pain, these methods place emphasis on proper technique and form in order to bring the body into alignment. By bringing the

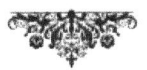

spine specifically into proper alignment, many symptoms of back pain can be relieved. Certain branches of chiropractic medicine and yoga also believe that bringing the spine into alignment can solve other health problems. According to these philosophies, because there are energy meridians or channels running along the spine, proper alignment allows for optimal flow - and therefore, ideal health - in all areas of life and the body.

Yoga's strong emphasis on not just the body, but the mind, is also theorized to be a huge help in the treatment of back pain. By quieting and controlling the mind, many things are possible. First, relaxation is widely known to have an impact on pain. Anxiety causes tension, and tension causes pain. Secondly, a conscious control of the mind can help greatly in managing pain by directing attention elsewhere. The pain may still be there, but you don't necessarily have to focus on it. Some have even claimed greater control of the mind has helped them consciously harness the placebo effect to help alleviate their pain.

Continuing education courses for yoga teachers have many directions to venture into. When considering the direction of one's yoga education, it might be worth

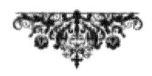

considering your student's needs. When we encounter so many people with back pain, it might be prudent to learn more yoga techniques that can help them.

YOGA IN PRACTICE - TEACHING YOGA WITH HUMILITY

Yoga has similarities to many other philosophies in regard to humility. However, Gurus and Swamis traditionally chose their students. In fact, much like traditional martial arts students, Yoga students traditionally saw training with their teacher as a privilege. Prospective students would seek out a Yoga teacher, begging to be accepted for instruction.

Now, we have the age of entitlement. No matter how many signs you put up, cell phones ring off in Yoga classes. No matter how many rules you have, a small number of students continue to break old rules and create new ones. If you hand the studio policies to a new student, you may hear, "Why do you have so many rules?"

After all, you posted them on the web site, your bulletin board, and now you take time for the orientation of each new student. Why do you have to explain each "for

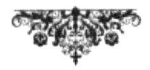

instance?" Sometimes, you may ask yourself, "What was my main objective, when I decided to become a Yoga teacher?"

Back to reality: Most of us decided to teach Yoga because we felt the positive benefits of a steady practice. As a result, we wanted to share the gift of Yoga instruction with others. Creating rules about taking a bath, taking your shoes off, and how to be respectful to others, is not part of what Yoga teacher intern's envision.

Then, one day, a new student shows up to class, but he may never have taken a bath in this lifetime. You may have read about this, but you have never been in the presence of an aroma like this before. Thoughts begin to run through your mind, and you are going to teach a class in ten minutes.

What exactly is that? You could speculate on how long that aroma has aged. What are you going to do? You have other students and this person is wearing "student repellant." This is surely a "lose-lose" situation. Do you have a rule made up for this?

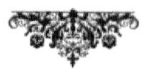

This is one situation, of many, in which your Yoga teacher training may not have prepared you. Sometimes, you may have to turn a student away. There is no need for conflict, if a student is not a "good fit;" you have the right to refuse to teach him or her.

This is much similar to the way students "shop around," if they do not like something about you, or your classes. You can be assertive without being guided by ego. Develop your skills to lead, motivate, and direct Yoga students, with compassion and tolerance.

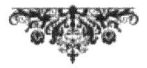

CHAPTER 16

7 TIPS ON HOW TO COMBINE YOGA AND WEIGHT TRAINING - ROUTINES THAT WILL SURELY BOOST YOUR WEIGHT LOSS

Did you know that you could now combine two extreme workouts to produce optimum results? In this chapter, we will tell you about the 7 tips on how to combine yoga and weight training perfectly. These routines will surely boost your weight loss so make sure to read this chapter from top to bottom.

As we all know, normal weight training requires a person to do three to five sets of one exercise. Each set comes with 8 to 12 repetitions of each exercise. Rest periods are important with each set finished giving your muscle time to recover and these periods last from 30 to 90 seconds only. They are essential parts of the workout, but we all know that they are the "down time" part of the program. The reason that we are paying attention to rest periods because some people spend more time resting than lifting weight, which is not recommended. With our 7 tips on how to combine yoga and weight training, you do not have

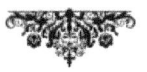

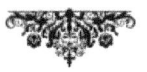

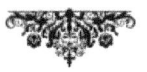87

to worry again with this problem because we will teach you how to mix power and grace with these two extreme workouts. Below are our 7 tips on how to combine yoga and weight training:

1. You need to think ahead with your routine. You have to determine how many sets of how many exercises you can do because this will serve as the framework of how to combine these workouts. You also need to know what poses you can do for the yoga, so we can incorporate it into the frame work.

2. Begin with your normal routine, which can be mild cardiovascular exercises or stretching. Let go of your worries during this time.

3. Finish one set of weight training exercise.

4. After finishing that, execute your first yoga pose for your rest period to avoid wasting time.

5. Do another set of your normal lift routine.

6. Follow it up with your pose for your rest period.

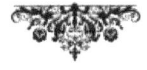

7. Continue to repeat steps three through six until you finish your workout.

Now you want to have more energy, be Healthier, look Younger, lose weight, and cleanse your body, right?
TEACHING YOGA: BECOME AN EXAMPLE OF MINDFULNESS

When you are mindful, you are alert and active. You recognize the thoughts coming in and out of your head, while noticing how your body is moving and feeling. Mindfulness is a total body and thought awareness that comes with deliberate consciousness. Mindfulness is an important part of Yoga practice because it allows you to let your thoughts come in and out, without focusing too heavily on any one thought. It allows you to be completely present as you move your body, stretch your muscles, and bring a fresh oxygen supply to your organs. Yoga instructors should always model mindfulness for their students.

When we spend too much time on any one thought or worry, it grows. The mind is a powerful tool for creating

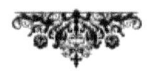

something rather large out of something possibly insignificant. Being mindful can help, because it allows us to take life one moment at a time. We can sit in the present moment and appreciate it for what it is. Mindfulness fosters gratitude and appreciation for all of the "small" things in life. Yoga is an opportunity to take a break from daily routines and stresses to be mindful of our bodies, our spirits, and our deeper purposes in life.

Yoga instructors can teach the concept of mindfulness during meditation practice. Students should sit or lie in a comfortable position, breathing deeply into the belly and chest. As the student's breathe, ask them to acknowledge each thought as it passes through their mind, then let it go. Guide the students to become aware of each part of their bodies, then move on to the next. Start with the toes and feet, move up to the calves, knees, and thighs. Keep traveling up the body, asking student's to acknowledge the body part, release and relax any tension, and move on. This exercise will help your student's learn to reach a state of mindfulness.

During Yoga class, instructors can remind students to be mindful by giving specific cues for each pose. Ask

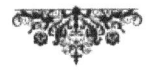

students to move specific parts of the body, and pay attention to how their bodies feel. Ask them to recognize any discomfort and adjust accordingly. Ask them to go deeper into the stretch, by breathing and feeling the moment, for exactly what it is. When Yoga teachers make a choice to consistently discuss, remind, and practice mindfulness, our students will begin to implement it into their own practices with ease.

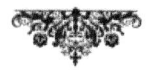

CHAPTER 17

TEACHING YOGA STUDENTS ABOUT THE
IMPORTANCE OF SLEEP

W hat is the value of Yoga Nidra (sleep of the Yogis)? Deep relaxation techniques, taught in Yoga classes, can become life savers outside the class. Although we should not take sleep period short cuts, Yoga Nidra is effective for bringing the mind and body to a state of rest, while the mind maintains awareness.

How many people wish they could work longer and get something accomplished instead of sleeping? How many times is the relaxation or meditation segment of a Yoga class taken for granted by students? Many will remark at how they feel a state of bliss or how mentally rested they feel after class.

Yet, how many students take their relaxation practice home? Very few Yoga students understand the benefits of relaxation and meditation. One way to drive the point

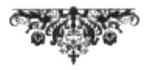

home is to design a pamphlet, or a flyer, which discusses the consequences of sleep deprivation and the benefits of relaxation.

Now is a time when many people work all day and night. They work at home, after they have left their jobs, and some have second or third jobs. Many people readily admit that when they wake up, they answer Email or do research on the Internet in the middle of their sleep cycle. After an hour or so, they go back to bed.

For some of us, broken sleep cycles do not bother us. However, some people really need a solid sleep cycle to function properly on the following day. Broken sleep sessions seem to work fine for my cats, but many humans tend to function better on eight solid hours of sleep.

The results of sleep deprivation are tricky. Each of us may respond with a slight difference. Some of the many symptoms, due to lack of sleep include: inability to concentrate, nervous behavior, irritability, sleeping during meetings, lack of motivation, reduced decision-making skills, and an appearance of tiredness.

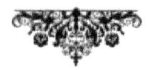

Worse still - sleep deprivation can cause automobile accidents, depression, and heart disease. The need to relax and sleep is a matter of survival. With that said, Yogic relaxation techniques are more than temporary rest, to be experienced once per week, in a Yoga class.

HOW IS HOT YOGA DIFFERENT FROM OTHER FORMS OF YOGA?

Customary forms of yoga have been practiced for more than five thousand years. Hot yoga is actually a fairly new type of yoga seeing that it has only emerged in the past fifty years.

Hot yoga is a phrase that identifies any variety of yoga routines carried out inside a warmed atmosphere.

The reason behind practising yoga inside of a hot place is to cause the entire body to perspire which assists the removing of toxins through your blood circulation and skin. Furthermore, it can provide a more enhanced, most beneficial routine since the warm temperature warms up the muscle tissues which makes them more workable and less vulnerable to accidental injury.

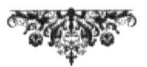

The temperature range of a particular hot yoga class room ranges somewhere between 30°C and 50°C (85°F to 122°F) for the practice, including a humidity level ranging from 40% to 60%.

There are more than just a single form of hot yoga, the most popular indeed being Bikram yoga. Bikram is so referred to because of its owner, Bikram Choudhury, who invented the method from the classic sort of Hatha yoga when he arrived in San Francisco in 1972.

In a move thought of by quite a few in the yoga community as a little egotistic, Bikram has branded his program. This program encompasses 26 positions and 2 breathing routines that are practiced in sequence, twice each during the 90 minute session. 45 minutes of this session is devoted to standing up postures and the additional 45 minutes is specifically for floor stances.

Versions of Hot Yoga

Bikram yoga is not the only form. Other kinds include The Barkan Method, Forrest yoga, power yoga, Core Power Yoga, Moksha yoga and Tribalance yoga. Here is a quick introduction to a few of these.

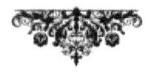

The Barkan Method of Hot Yoga was established in 2002 by Jimmy Barkan, a trainee of Bikram Choudhury. Barkan's technique is in line with the teachings of Bikram's yet it involves positions from other kinds of yoga and doesn't stick to a permanent collection of poses. Unlike Bikram, Barkan incorporates a vinyasa motion within his classes - a set of interrelated stances that can be coordinated together with the respiration.

Forrest yoga was established in the 1980s by Ana T. Forrest. Its objective is on psychological and bodily re-conditioning. It helps and really encourages people to look at how much they understand about their body on the mat and draw it into their day to day life.

Moksha yoga is a variety of hot yoga which was set up by Ted Grant together with Jessica Robertson in Toronto, Canada in 2004. This method is dedicated to the availability of the practice and thinks that yoga is for all people. Furthermore, it has dedicated eco-friendly and sustainability guidelines which are generally applicable to each of the Moksha yoga studios across the globe.

Tribalance yoga is another version of hot yoga with a program more or less the opposite of Bikram yoga. As for instance, the classes require dim light sources to make a more inner journey within the pupil, which is unlike Bikram yoga, in which bright lights are a regulation.

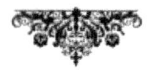

CHAPTER 18

TEACHING YOGA FOR HAPPINESS

Think back to a time of no responsibility, with a wide-eyed view of life and reality. When we were kids, how many of my friends said, "When I grow up, I'm going to become a Yoga teacher?" If memory serves me right, the answer is: "None."

Now, let's fast forward to the present. Most of us were absorbed into the corporate world. Maybe some of us resisted joining "The Establishment," for a while, but eventually most of us settled down to raise families and go to work.

Like our parents and grandparents, some of us worked for Fortune 500 companies, which would "take care of you for life." We may have believed that myth, but economics, recessions, and lay offs, bring about a new reality.

It seems that economies expand and contract, approximately, every seven to ten years. Any sort of economic downturn can become a financial disaster for the individuals and families that are affected by it. How can anyone be happy, when they are unemployed?

Happiness is sometimes associated with our personal viewpoint of control. We wish to control our lives, but we have limits. So, what can you do to brace for the ebb and flow of changing economies? Whether we like it, or not, we are all "free agents." Employers must do what is necessary to keep their companies alive.

For each of us, this means part-time employment, or part-time self-employment, doing something that will help your family make ends meet. This opens the door for many options, including becoming a Yoga instructor.

There has always been a belief in the "All or Nothing" theory. For example, some will tell you: "Become a full-time Yoga teacher, or don't do it at all." Firstly, most teachers of Yoga start out part-time. So, why listen to nonsense?

It takes time to establish yourself in any field. Why should anyone think he or she should take the plunge with "both feet first?" The most conservative way to start teaching Yoga sessions is by becoming an independent contractor or by teaching at a garage, loft, barn, or basement.

In this way, you are not taking any financial risks and you learn so much more by teaching. As a part-time Yoga teacher, you learn about people, ailments, and how not to

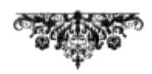

waste your time or money. You will continue to educate yourself for life and you will find true happiness.

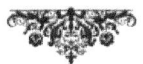

EIGHT AMAZING BENEFITS OF TEACHING YOGA:

Every challenging occupation yields some sort of satisfaction, but the fitness professional's industry had an amazing 85% job satisfaction rate according to an Idea Health & Fitness survey.

Job Satisfaction

In the same survey, 98% of those interviewed felt that "My work gives me a feeling of personal accomplishment." Lack of personal satisfaction is the most frequent reason why people leave a job. These statistics make it obvious that this is an extremely harmonious atmosphere to work in.

For many of us who worked in the corporate world and shifted into the health and fitness industry, the energy felt in a health club, ashram, or wellness center is similar to being on vacation. There's always something to do, but the job itself is very gratifying.

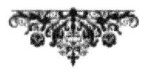

Rewards of Helping Family, Friends, Students, and Co-workers

Your self esteem improves as you find solutions for the pain management of others, ailments, fitness, stress management, positive thinking, etc.

The list goes on, as you continue your own journey of self improvement, but the feeling of gratification you get from helping someone find the right path, is beyond words.

You will always remember: That student who reaches their ideal body weight, the physically impaired student who finds that they, too, can live a better quality life, and the student who leaves your class without the headache or backache they came in with.

Your Own Health

As a practitioner of Yoga, you have become more aware of your daily ups and downs. You monitor your breath, posture, moods, diet, and exercise on a daily basis.

As a Yoga teacher, you are setting an example to your students and teaching them to live a quality life. This path will enable you to live longer and live better.

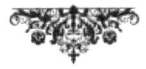

There is no Shortage of Work

When the working world is in the "9 to 5" mode, you have many opportunities with Corporate Accounts, The Fitness Industry, Senior Centers, Medical Centers, Referrals, etc. This is when you to teach them, with any free time you have.

The object is to contact them. This is where your post cards come in handy, if you don't have a personal referral.

Continuing Education

Yes, learning new things keeps your mind stimulated and healthy. You will never tire of subject's to study, explore, and investigate. There are so many facets of Yoga, that one life span, is just not enough time to learn it all.

It's not a race, but it is a journey. You will find friends, colleagues, and students who are on the same path. This makes giving, receiving, and sharing a wonderful thing along the way.

Time

You will have time to stop, think, breathe, relax, or meditate. You can always fill your plate beyond its limits, but you no longer have to.

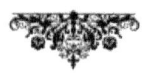

You can determine whether or not you will be stuck in traffic during rush hour. You decide what hours you will work and what days you have off. You will come to the realization that your time is your own.

Independence

Everyone wants control of their own life, but very few achieve it. Being in business for yourself, can help you control your own destiny and that of your family.

Sure there are limits to what one person can accomplish, but it is better to try than to have never tried.

Success

No matter what you want, if you write down your short-term and long-term goals, you will make great progress toward them.

You should keep these goals in a place where you can see them daily and visualize yourself accomplishing your goals. You should be specific about time frames and ethical methods used to meet them. You can even use them in meditation.

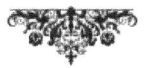

Review your long-term goals at least once every season and every year. Review your short-term goals daily. You will see yourself make rapid success in this way.

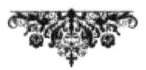

CHAPTER 19

MASTERING THE CRAFT OF TEACHING YOGA

Did you ever question your devotion to teaching Yoga? Have you ever internally questioned the devotion of another Yoga teacher? It is only human to question and make comparisons. Making comparisons, and judging, has kept you alive up to this point. Every step in life requires you to make some form of judgment or a decision.

You can freely decide to become a Yoga teacher. You decide whether to get out of bed, or not, each day. You choose to eat breakfast, take a shower, meditate, watch television, or anything else, after you wake up. To choose, or decide, is a form of judgment. So, how did we get the idea that judgment should be restrained?

Our judgments, and pre-conceived notions, concerning ourselves and others, can be self-destructive. Prejudice and intolerance have led humankind toward the path of hate, and narrow-minded thinking, throughout history. We have also learned that harsh judgments of others hold us back as a species.

This is why non-judgment is praised as a higher quality. Tolerance and mutual respect, over our differences, gives us the power of collective thinking. When we communicate with others, who have different thoughts; we collectively learn from the experience. This ability, to accept differences in others, is the path to progress for humankind.

Due to Internet communication, television, and radio, we have access to new ideas every day. This does not mean all outside ideas will be easily accepted, but we have come a long way since our cave dwelling ancestors. New ideas are subject to practical application and time. This is why any fresh ideas are worthy of "air time."

In judging ourselves too harshly, we waste time wishing we could change the past. This is a mistake that can lead to feelings of regret, depression, and self-contempt. The experience from mistakes, helps us learn more about what we are made of. We are better off to learn from our past mistakes, try to correct them, and move forwar - enriched by the experience.

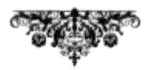

Many interns join Yoga teacher training courses as a quest for self-discovery. The journey of understanding your true purpose in life is a noble path, but it is not the end of the path. If you are lucky enough to understand yourself, and you know your unique purpose in this life, you should help others who are seeking answers.

TEACHING YOGA TO BUILD STRENGTH

When you decided to become a yoga instructor, did you think you would get so many different requests? Many women and men want to gain strength without gaining size. As we know, more size is stressful on the leg joints and the heart. As a yoga instructor your mission is to help people maintain a long and healthy life.

As most lifelong yogis will explain, the original purpose of practicing yoga was not physical fitness or weight loss; rather, yoga is a spiritual discipline that uses increased connection with the physical body to achieve personal transcendence. Since the rapid proliferation of yoga studios all over the world over the last two decades, however, yoga has undergone a modernization wherein some of the most popular forms of yoga are practiced as exercise, rather than as a spiritual practice.

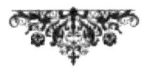

The reasons why a spiritual discipline has been transformed into a mostly physical one are numerous, but it is nearly certain that yoga probably would not have become so popular if it were not for advantages of firming the body, strength building, increased flexibility and aerobic improvements. Yoga instructors soon realized that advocating a yogic lifestyle as a tool for better health and fitness would attract a variety of practitioners.

Yoga does build strength. As beginners know, many of the poses are difficult to hold and muscles can begin to quake early on in a yoga session. As muscles fatigue and continue to work, they undergo a process where they are broken down and then built back up during rest periods. This makes the body stronger.

Tips for Teaching Yoga to Build Strength

1. Remind students to be patient. While weight training typically isolates muscle groups and allows individuals to bulk up and see results relatively quickly, yoga practice builds strength via body weight lifts and holds. In other words, the weight a yoga student lifts is his or her own,

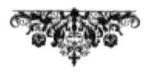

and this can take longer than a typical weight lifting routine to build strength because it is a slower approach designed to improve physical health over time.

2. Keep the flow fast so muscles will have less time to recover after a challenging pose. This will ensure that muscle group's tire quicker and thus have to work harder in yoga poses.

3. As students progress in yoga, instructor's can adapt a series of movements by encouraging students to hold poses longer and do more repetitions. Doing more repetitions means that yogis will work the same muscle group's harder during a single yoga session, building more strength and endurance than they would with fewer repetitions.

4. Focus on balance, inversion and standing poses to build the most strength. Remember that a yoga series should strengthen the body in balance instead of isolating legs one day and doing arms the next, which is the standard practice of weight-lifting routines.

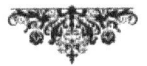

CHAPTER 20

WHY GETTING YOGA TEACHER TRAINING ONLINE
IS THE BEST ROUTE FOR GETTING CERTIFIED

Becoming a Yoga teacher can be not only a profitable career, but it could allow for oneself to achieve amazing flexibility and share their knowledge with others. The Yoga industry is growing every year with more studios opening up and more programs to teach future instructors. One of the newest forms of programs is the Yoga teacher training online where they allow for potential teachers to get certified online.

Why The Yoga Industry Is Booming

Yoga is constantly growing in many places. Countless people are trying to get fit and stay healthy, and they are heading down to Yoga classes to supplement their gym time. Yoga has studios in dozens of countries and states, and more people are getting certified. Not only is the career outlook going to last for many more years, but the need and the development of more Yoga studios enables

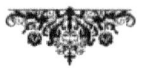

for more instructors to be in more demand later down the road.

Is Being A Yoga Teacher A Profitable Career?

Being an instructor can mean many hours of work in a many studios. An instructor could earn several hundred by the end of the day teaching as an employed instructor, but even more in their own studio. The opportunities are endless for Yoga instructors.

Why Getting Yoga Teacher Training Online Is The Best Route

Any person wanting to become a teacher would know that they need to work hours and hours every single week to perfect the craft of Yoga to the best of their ability in order to one day teach. It is common for some people to get as many hours of Yoga training in a professional studio just to learn the concept of Yoga and get a good basis for it. To teach, a person must spend a certain amount of hours learning and receiving a specific amount of training to be certified.

It is the best route to go online because it allows for the instructor to learn from home. It saves time, energy, and

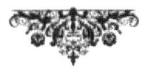

112

money to learn from the Internet, and it provides the opportunity to improve technique and learn from his or herself. As an instructor, learning to make critiques to oneself is an amazing skill.

What Is Involved In Online Yoga Training

The Yoga practitioner will learn about correct Yoga form, and how as a teacher, one could find those mistakes in their students. They'll discover the correct techniques for becoming not just a great Yoga teacher, but a great Yoga student themselves. It is vital for the instructor to know the proper way to showcase Yoga poses and discover the easy version of poses to help their students, and it is all taught in the training.

Certification is given when a person completes the training. Usually, there is going to be a time for a certified instructor to see the trained Yoga practitioner to make sure they are truly capable of teaching a class. The training provides users with all the guidance needed to ensure they are prepared to get their certification and receive the chance to start teaching this amazing form of exercise.

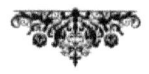

THREE METHODS FOR TEACHING YOGA STUDENTS HOW TO CULTIVATE POSITIVE ENERGY

Students often attend Yoga sessions for relief from a constant barrage of negative messages during the day. If you listen to the news for ten minutes, you are likely to feel puzzled as to why so much social injustice still exists. Anyone can change the world for the best, by cultivating positive energy, and teaching others how to do the same thing.

Just like anything else, cultivation of positive energy requires a plan of action; otherwise, we will spend the vast majority of the day reacting to bad news. One method is to visualize and plan the day ahead. Some people feel they have no control over their lives. In fact, they do not have control over their lives because they have envisioned it.

Visualize Tomorrow

This requires a little time on the night before, but it is much similar to packing your lunch for the next day. Another way to make visualization more real is to write down your tasks and objective, while allowing some time for the unexpected surprises that life gives us.

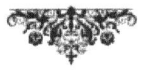

Avoid Energy Drains

Unfortunately, there are people who sap energy from everyone else. One person I know refers to them as "time bandits." They manage to fill the day with self-created obstacles, engage in lengthy pessimistic conversations, or talk about the flaws everyone else has.

You could compare them to human land mines. You can be hurt, the longer you spend time with them. You feel the energy being sapped away from you as their list of grievances grows. You may have tried to help before, but their goal is to complain about everything.

In reality, you choose who you associate with. If you associate with someone who drains your energy, you have to make some decisions to improve your life, or stay in a life boat with an energy drainer, drifting aimlessly through oceans of pessimism.

It is not easy to turn your back on anyone. However, if you show someone there is light at the end of the tunnel, and they refuse to see it, you have to move forward or allow someone else to hold you back.

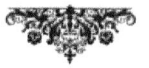

Define Your True Self

In Yoga, we learn to identify one's true self. Some call the cosmic self: "atma." We also learn to avoid judging ourselves and others harshly. It is true that we are not our thoughts, but our thoughts have a way of defining us - in the form of self-criticism, regret, and negative thoughts.

Yoga teaches us to honestly look inside, to see the good and the bad. We can change today for a better tomorrow, but we cannot change anything until we stop engaging in self-criticism.

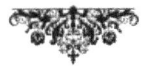

CHAPTER 21

WHY TEACHING VINYASA YOGA ROCKS

Yoga is becoming increasingly popular as a way to stay in shape and increase happiness. People of all ages enjoy classes and the benefits that this practice provides. Teaching vinyasa yoga in particular provides flowing techniques that increase flexibility, build muscle, and release endorphins. As a result, yoga makes you happier, healthier, and stronger. Imagine if your job involved this great practice? As an instructor, you can enjoy a job that provides many benefits that other careers simply do not have.

Here are the many reasons teaching vinyasa yoga rocks:

Your Job Keeps You in Shape

Say goodbye to sitting at a desk, typing away all day long. This lack of activity is draining and unhealthy. As an instructor, you are able to stay in shape while working at the same time! Instead of leaving work feeling like you have gained ten pounds from sitting all day, you will leave work feeling refreshed and healthy!

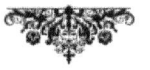

Plus, as with all exercise, you release endorphins which are chemicals that have shown to increase mood. So, as an instructor, your job will literally make you feel happier! What more could you want from a career?

You Will Meet Great People

People attend classes because it makes them happy. Imagine if everyone at work was there because they were happy to be there. That's what it is like when you teach vinyasa yoga! You will meet great people who all have a motivation to keep themselves happy and healthy. It is a great place to connect with people who have similar interests and values as you.

You Gain an Appreciation for Life

Much of yoga is about bettering your life. It provides an opportunity for people to slow down, take a deep breath, and focus on happiness. The breathing techniques in the practice are meant to create peace and happiness within yourself.

Did you know that you learn best when you teach something? So, if you lead yoga, you will become an

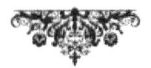

expert at focusing on happy thoughts and appreciating the moment. You will learn how to be great at blocking our negative thoughts and enjoying the little things that make life great.

Your Job is a Constant Motivator

As an instructor, you are encouraging others to practice techniques that keep them healthy and strong. You will be helping individuals make a better life for themselves by adopting healthy lifestyle techniques. In doing so, you will be constantly reminding yourself of the importance of this lifestyle too! After all, we all must practice what we teach, right?

If you are looking for a career that makes you feel great and keeps you healthy, than teaching vinyasa is a perfect job. Instead of wasting away at a desk all day long throw on a tank top and hit the yoga studio so you can begin working towards a career that is completely awesome.

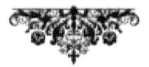

CHAPTER 22

WHY CHAIR YOGA

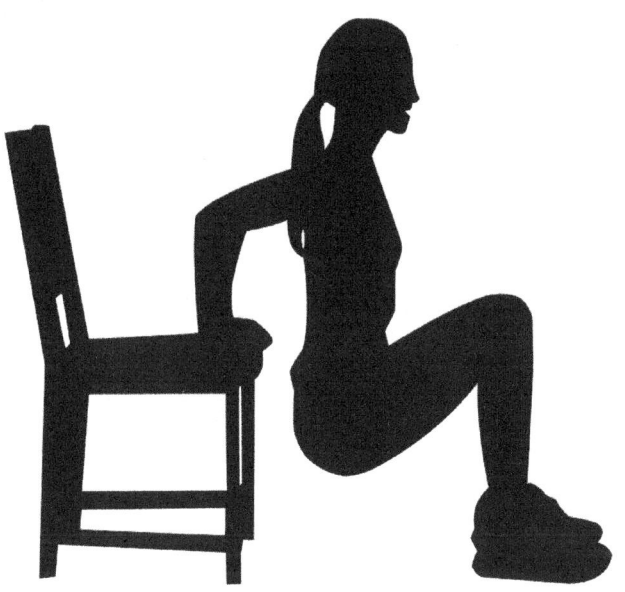

Isn't Yoga just for young "hard bodies," like you would see on the cover of a magazine? Don't you have to turn your body into a pretzel, to practice Yoga? These are, a few of the many, questions i am asked about Yoga and Chair Yoga. Any idea that Yoga is only for the fit, and young, is a complete myth. Anyone can practice Yoga, at any age, but not all Yoga styles are the same.

Many of us struggle, most of our lives, to find the optimum exercise routine, in order to stay in shape. As time goes by, we look for low-impact fitness solutions, due to excessive wear in our joints. It can't be helped that, joints will wear, as our bodies take a lifetime of stress, tumbles, and injuries.

Low-impact exercise philosophy works like this: "No pain - No gain," slogans are definitely short-term thinking. When you consider longevity, you want to receive maximum benefits, of a health maintenance program, without abusing or unnecessarily wearing, any body parts out.

It is far better to intelligently exercise the body, than to work the body hard with risk of injury. To injure oneself, while exercising, is irony in its purest form. After all, isn't the purpose of exercise to improve or maintain your health?

So, the one reason to try a Yoga class is because you have found a low-impact exercise solution. Chair Yoga will develop or maintain the body's circulation, flexibility and

strength, with very low impact. It is a complete health maintenance exercise program.

There is also the social factor. It's good to get out of the house and socialize with friends and family members in a different setting. In fact, Chair Yoga is just one of many activities that take place in the average senior center. You can usually find dancing, Tai Chi, various exercise programs, crafts, card games, and many more activities, in the average senior center.

Back to Chair Yoga: It goes by a variety of different names and is sometimes mixed with other forms of exercise, within the same class, such as: weight resistance, low-impact aerobics, Chair Pilates.

Some of the many names associated with these classes are: Stretch, Stretch and Tone, Senior Yoga, Wellness, and Senior Fitness. As mentioned before these classes may contain a mixture of low-impact exercises from different origins.

There is also, another reason to start a Chair Yoga class. What if you suddenly found your mobility limited or were

confined to a wheel chair? A common belief is that, Chair Yoga is only for seniors. As you already know, limited mobility has nothing to do with age, and can be a problem, at any point in life.

FIVE REASONS FOR YOGA INSTRUCTORS TO TEACH CHAIR YOGA:

1) Your students truly benefit from it.

Your students will likely be either seniors or those with physical limitations. Especially in the case of someone that has not been exercising at all because of their condition, you will often see rapid improvements. Prospective students sometimes report feeling better after a single class.

2) Your work will be truly appreciated and you'll hear about it, too.

You will often enjoy having people tell you about all the wonderful things that chair yoga has done to make them more comfortable, healthier, and happier.

Those of us that are younger and don't have a debilitating condition tend to take some things for granted. Chair yoga

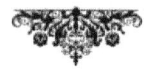

might help a person raise their arm above their heads to reach something, or turn their head back to check traffic, when they had lost the ability to do so. I think I'd be appreciative, too!

3) Millions of prospective students and growing daily.
So much has been said about the value of marketing into the coming boom in baby boomer seniors that i shouldn't have to convince you. Besides, we can all see it happening right before our very eyes.

As a yoga instructor, adding chair yoga to your list of teaching skills is a good way to take advantage of this social phenomenon.

Baby boomers aren't much interested in retiring to sit back in a rocking chair and wait while their bodies deteriorate from disuse. So no matter what age or stage they are in, they will be seeking ways to keep themselves fit.

Baby boomers are more likely to consider alternate approaches to staying healthy than previous generations, so they will be much more likely to be receptive to the

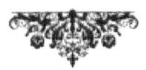

124

notion of practicing yoga. In fact, many will have some sort of prior experience with yoga, as we have seen.

The oldest of the boomers are just now turning 60, so it is a great time to get serious about teaching chair yoga!

4) There is an abundance of ready-made classes to find.

Most yoga classes come about in an organic fashion, adding one or two students at a time. But by teaching chair yoga, you can find yourself starting whole new classes with several customers all at once.

This is because you are often taking the yoga class to the people where they are already congregating. One of the biggest markets for chair yoga is seniors, and seniors are easy to find already in a group together.

Just where to go will vary depending on where you live, but here are a few ideas to get you started thinking about this:

> ➢ Retirement villages, retirement centers, assisted living centers, nursing homes

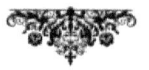

- Adult day care
- Seniors' groups at places of worship
- Community centers/Parks and recreation programs
- Fraternal organizations
- Libraries
- YMCA/YWCA

People suffering from particular ailments such as multiple sclerosis or arthritis tend to get together to help each other cope with the disease. All you have to do is find the organizations in your neighborhood that are addressing this need and approach them with the idea of helping the group practice chair yoga. Yoga has been shown to effectively ease the symptoms of many types of ailments, and yet few have anyplace to go where there is a yoga program appropriate for them.

With some brainstorming you can probably come up with a pretty good list appropriate for the circumstances in your community.

The beauty of approaching these groups is that you almost always are proposing to teach yoga to people that never imagined they'd be in a yoga class. That means you aren't

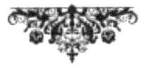

competing with all the yoga teachers trying to capture classes out of the existing pool of practicing yogis and yoginis.

Just how you go about approaching these types of organizations is something that we go into detail about in our Yoga in Chairs teacher training intensives and the materials for the at-home training program.

5) Enjoy having loyal students.

There are many reasons why chair yoga students will be more loyal to you than students in your more traditional classes.

It is likely that they were introduced to yoga by you or by the leadership of the group they are in. Since they never had a notion to seek out yoga before, they will be much less inclined to look for alternative teachers in your area. Plus, as has already been noted, they probably don't have many other chair yoga programs to turn to, even if they wanted to have choices.

If you take the class to the students it is of course easy for them to participate every time you are there.

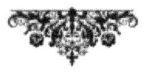

Most of your chair yoga customers will be mature people who know the value of being considered reliable. This means that when they make a commitment to participate in a program, they likely will follow through.

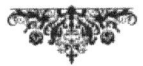

CHAPTER 23

FIVE REASONS STUDENTS STOP COMING TO YOGA CLASS

Every Yoga teacher has experienced it: a new student comes to practice, and he or she seems to do well. They never ask a question or for clarification, but after a practice, they disappear. What happened?

Five reasons why students stop coming to Yoga class, and what Yoga teachers can do about it:

1) The class is comprised of mixed levels, and the student finds the practice either too easy or too difficult.

Ideally, Yoga is about challenging oneself and perfecting one's own practice; realistically, students enjoy practice with others of a similar level. The challenge for an instructor is offering quality to every student, even if they have diverse needs. Some of the ways to help include acknowledging the nature of a mixed level class is making a statement, such as, "We have some people here today

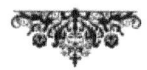

who have been practicing for quite some time, and others who are new to the practice. I'll demonstrate the full asana first, and a modification afterwards; please work at your own level," can go a long way toward making all practitioners feel accepted. If the class is large, consider scheduling a beginner and an advanced class, rather than mixed level.

2) The student felt that the class was too expensive.

Make sure that a variety of payment options are available, if at all possible. Multi-class punch cards, student discounts, and a community class are all ways that studios and teachers can make classes accessible. As a practitioner advances, he or she is more likely to see higher cost classes as an investment, and be willing to pay full price.

3) The Yoga class was uncomfortable.

Be certain that the space you will be teaching in is clean, quiet, and reasonably cool. If the class is full, take the initiative in asking students to re-arrange mats to accommodate everyone. Many people feel uncomfortable asking others to move their mats and appreciate the Yoga instructor stepping in to help. Alternatively, the

atmosphere may not have been as nurturing as hoped. Did many Yoga students arrive late or get up and leave during Savasana? Consider speaking privately to "repeat offenders," who do not respect the length of the class.

4) The style of Yoga was not what they expected.

Be sure class descriptions and starting times are clear and up-to-date, to the extent you are able, with the studio or website. Indicate whether it will be a gentler Hatha Yoga or a vigorous Ashtanga practice, and consider including the information in your introduction at the beginning of class.

5) The Yoga class has diversity issues.

In a class full of middle-aged, or older, Yoga students, a college student may not feel comfortable. Practitioners with disabilities may not want to "stand out" during practice, and students who are heavier may feel as if they are under scrutiny for their weight. If you, as a Yoga instructor, truly believe that Yoga is for everyone, be sure that your attitude reflects acceptance of those who differ in age, race, gender, or size. While you do not control who attends the class, you set the tone for the group, and should be certain that it is welcoming to all.

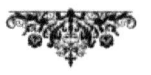

CHAPTER 24

YOGA FOR PREVENTION AND TERMINATION OF DRUG ABUSE

Yoga, as well as other alternative therapies, has been practiced for the purpose of ending drug abuse with fair results. Many people ask how Yoga helps people quit abusing drugs. The Yogic method for ending substance abuse is very simple. Yoga gives the mind a useful daily purpose, which re-programs the practitioner.

Drugs fill a void in the mind and body. Even though we disagree with drug abuse, it must be noted that drugs either stimulate or dull the senses. This is one of the main reasons, why someone would try drugs in the first place.

Whether it is physical or mental, drug addiction is a result of habit. This habit had to be formed because the addict found the experience pleasurable. Many drug addicts feel they have nothing to live for, and they are not thinking about living for longevity.

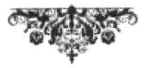

In terms of holistic health, drug addiction is the exact opposite of all forms of Yoga. Yoga is a discipline based upon developing, and maintaining, optimum health. Serious Yoga practitioners tend to eliminate substances, which can be abused, because they do not need them.

Yoga already stimulates the mind and body, but for the purpose of improving the practitioner's health. This is where Yoga could save humanity from drug abuse. Instead of focusing on the "Drug War," why not teach Yoga, to children, globally?

Yoga programs for children would prevent drug abuse and eliminate the need for stimulating, or dulling, and the senses. In one generation, we could eliminate the need for illegal drugs and the crimes related to them.

Yoga practice does not have any harmful side effects. A drug addict, who wants to quit, will benefit from Pranayama (Yogic breathing techniques), Asana (Yoga Postures), Meditation, and many more aspects that Yoga has to offer.

HOW YOGA TEACHERS CAN ATTRACT MORE MEN TO YOGA CLASSES

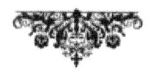

In India Yoga participation by men is ideal. Sadly, in some parts of the world, we teach Yoga classes primarily to a female audience. While women still outnumber men in many western Yoga studios, there are signs that this wonderful practice is becoming more readily accepted by the opposite gender. Endorsements by professional athletes and celebrities have helped to spread the word, but more education is needed before its feminine mystique becomes equally recognized as a manly endeavor.

To analyze why western males have difficulty staying in Yoga classes is a mystery to many. It seems that if one gender is in the minority, in regard to any activity, it is hard to reach out to that group. As a woman, I have seen the same in martial arts, boxing, and football, which are dominated by male participation.

Reaching Out

Just as Yoga has been marketed in recent years to target diverse groups, there are also ways to promote the practice among the male population. Like other sectors, not all men will respond to the same style of exercise or studio, but the good thing about Yoga is that it can be tailored to suit a wide spectrum of interests and participants.

The first step to attracting men is getting their attention, and the second is following through with a program that meets their individual needs.

Five Tips to Get Men Interested in Yoga:

1. Create classes that incorporate familiar skills, such as core work or martial arts, which put men at ease and allow them to see results.

2. Offer class options that provide the stamina and training needed to improve performance in other activities, such as weight lifting, football, golf, tennis or biking.

3. Emphasize the gender-specific ways that Yoga benefits men's health and reduces the likelihood of injuries in other areas.

4. Network. Hand out brochures, go to health fairs, or hold special events to let men in the community know about Yoga classes and what they can gain from them. Include testimonials from satisfied students or coupons for introductory offers on flyers and websites.

5. Ask students to tell their friends, husbands, and families about special offerings for men and provide incentives to those who bring in new students.

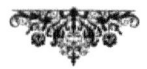

CHAPTER 25

YOGA OFF THE MAT - THREE YOGIC PRINCIPLES
FOR ACHIEVEMENT

The concept of deriving achievement from Yoga practice is nothing new. Yoga has the ability to alter anyone's direction in life. Throughout history, it has been possible to reach mental, emotional, physical, spiritual, and financial goals by practicing or teaching Yoga.

The debate over whether achievement is good, or not, and depends upon what we do with an opportunity. If one makes great financial achievements, and contributes large donations to charity, is that wrong? If one becomes a magnet of mental power, but uses it toward negatively manipulating students, is that right?

Common sense tells you that some people make the most of an opportunity, while some people will waste the same good fortune. Most people will not recognize an opportunity, and many more will not take action toward a successful outcome.

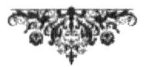

1. Karma: It is often said, that only 5% of those who have an opportunity will act on it. That is why the first method of achievement is action (karma). The actions we take, or fail to take, determine our path in life. We can change our course at any time.

However, our actions should be beneficial to those around us. If we are promoting, or enhancing well-being, this is a just cause. At the same time, any cause or action you take should be something for which you have a true passion. In this way, you will see your actions through, and complete your mission.

2. Transcendental Thought: Limited thinking holds most of us back, but transcendental thought encourages each of us to go far beyond what is expected. It is easy to criticize everything, but the mind works very hard to come up with possible solutions.

The answer to reducing your work is to listen to outside opinions. When we rationally consider the positive and negative opinions of others - there is usually a logical solution buried within the mixture of information. The

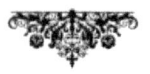

hard part is to extract information with impartial judgment.

3. Faith: To have faith in oneself is very powerful. To have faith, in the power of prayer, is also very powerful. It does not matter what your religion is, because the answers to your spiritual growth are within your religion. Too much time and energy is wasted on fighting over differences.

YOGA TEACHER CHRONICLES - YOGIC METHODS FOR DIFFUSING A CONFLICT

How can Yoga help us maintain our composure during a potential argument? The following Yogic methods are designed to help anyone keep their cool in the worst of times. We know that losing our temper in business, family, or public matters, tend to hurt relationships and prevent successful outcomes. So, let's look at some solutions to diffuse conflicts.

Learn to recognize the "triggers," which make you feel defensive or angry. This can be performed through careful observation of yourself and others. Carefully practice mindfulness each day, and observe yourself without

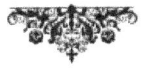

criticism. In life, we tend to be our own worst critics. Self-observation has nothing to do with self-criticism.

Self-observation is an honest view of your daily life, as it is. Once you see the truth and document it, then you can take action to alter it. Although, you have been taught the principles of Santosha (contentment), and you should be happy for what you have, you have the ability to make changes.

There is also a Sanskrit word: "Sankalpa," which means resolution. This is not the common shallow promise, which is made on January 1st, and disappears by Valentine's Day. This is a vow to perform a particular practice for a specific length of time. The act of observing, documenting, and taking corrective action, to diffuse conflicts, is a noble path, and full of gratification.

Through this method, some people completely learn to shut anger out of communication. For example: If a person is having a bad day, and makes an accusation toward you, he or she is often caught off guard, when you try to understand their point.

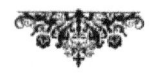

Empathic listening skills are rare, but the best diplomats have practiced and learned them well. If you are rational, and stick to the point of the conflict, by asking sincere, concerned questions about why someone is upset, you will sometimes resolve the conflict before it can escalate.

When you stop, and repeat what someone says, you demonstrate concern about the issues. At the same time, you show respect because you are pondering his or her point. This also prevents side issues, by maintaining focus on the main point of contention.

Lastly, if something makes you upset, and you need to "cool down," you should not be negotiating. It is human nature to have mind clutter. We practice, or teach Yoga, to organize the mind. Most of us cannot maintain a focused mind all the time.

With that said, there is a proper time and place for negotiations. Choose your "ground," make composure your ally, show poise, and then resolve conflicts peacefully.

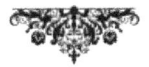

CHAPTER 26

FIVE REASONS WHY YOU SHOULD NOT BE A

YOGA TEACHER

Truthfully, there are no reasons why any of us cannot be, or do, what we want, as long as you are not hurting anyone. You should always strive to be the best you can be. However, you may find that many people create obstacles, in front of themselves, to avoid success.

This is truly ironic that we hold ourselves back from making achievements, and teaching Yoga is just one of many goals that are not fully realized. Below is a list of common reasons why many good Yoga practitioners do not pursue their goal of becoming a Yoga instructor.

"I am too old to teach Yoga."

Actually, age is not a factor. There are many styles of Yoga; and the most common, outside of India, is Hatha Yoga and its many sub-styles. Although Hatha Yoga is the

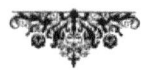

Union of physical mastery, it has many gentle and vigorous styles.

There is a need for mature, passionate, safety conscious, and gentle Yoga teachers. The world's population is aging and Yoga students are living longer. Who would have thought that hospitals and religious centers would seek out Yoga teachers ten or twenty years ago?

Therefore, Yoga is becoming readily accepted by mainstream society and does not have to apply to any one particular religious group. Some of the old barriers that prevented the masses from being exposed to Yoga are gone.

"Dancers, Martial Artists, and Gymnasts perform better Yoga asanas than I can."

Yoga is not dance, martial arts, or gymnastics. This is not to take away the importance of any of the above-mentioned arts. After all, I am a martial artist, and I was originally introduced to Yoga in a martial arts setting.

Being a little more flexible than the average person is a gift. However, it doesn't serve as a top priority for

teaching Yoga. The best Yoga teachers are those who can communicate, and those teachers usually have to struggle to excel at Yoga.

Yoga teachers who are naturally flexible think that everyone else should be, as well. This is not always the case, as there are skeletal limitations within some Yoga students. This is not to say that they cannot increase, or improve, their flexibility, but each person's body is unique.

"Teaching Yoga costs too much money."

This is true in some cases; however, you can shop around for the best course at the most affordable price. Some onsite Yoga training facilities have Seva Programs, where you can work for partial tuition. This is much like a college, where there are scholarships for students who perform tasks around the campus. There are also a variety of Yoga correspondence courses, which allow flexible study hours, little or no travel, and no extra expenses. My wellness center offers such a Yoga course, and we have interns and graduates worldwide.

"I only want to teach Yoga to a few students and I don't want to go into the Yoga business."

Many Yoga practitioners feel this way and that's fine. This is not a problem because if you are teaching a few friends, as a hobby, it is not necessary to go through the certification process.

If your circle of friends starts to expand, it would be wise to get some type of liability coverage. There are a number of liability insurance programs to choose. You could purchase a sports, Yoga, or home liability policy to cover your specific needs.

You should also learn as much as you can about safety, anatomy, physiology, and kinesiology. The reason I mention this is so that you do not hurt your Yoga students. The compassion and knowledge to become a safe Yoga instructor is very important.

"I have a good paying job and teaching Yoga may not support my family."

Like all start up small businesses Yoga cannot offer "instant bundles of cash." You would want to build your

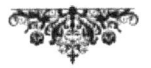

business as an independent contractor first. In our Yoga teacher course, you will find 16 ways to grow your business, with little or no overhead. When you build up enough accounts, the decision, as to whether or not to open your own independent Yoga studio, will be clear.

This has been a radical job change for all of us, who go into teaching Yoga full time, but you do not have to take any sudden or financial risks. Growing your own Yoga business can start on a part time basis and later develop into full time, if you get the right guidance and take the proper steps.

Bear in mind that the business and marketing information in our Yoga course is current and "field tested." This information is specific to Yoga instructors and contains successful methods used, with regard to return on investment.

Right now, there are a lot of Yoga studios that "flounder" economically, because the owners have insufficient business or marketing skills. Within this kind of climate, it is not hard to get your market share of Yoga students within your geographic area.

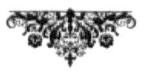

Lastly, there are so many reasons to avoid progress, you could create a book of excuses, but the reason to succeed at anything is your passion. If you are passionate, safe, and knowledgeable about Yoga, this is an excellent starting point for anyone who wants to become a Yoga teacher.

3 CHARACTERISTICS OF A BAD YOGA TEACHER

We're all human. I really believe that most yoga teachers don't have the intentions of doing harm to anyone or teaching yoga without having proper experience. Most of them have good intentions. But just like everyone else, they too may have bad days sometimes. And it's also a fact that even the greatest teachers start as inexperienced and beginner's who are finding their voices. So even if your teacher has one or two of these characteristics, it doesn't mean he/she can't teach you anything. However, you should proceed with caution.

Here are some less-desirable characteristics of a yoga teacher:

1. He knows everything. The flip side of an unsure teacher is the teacher who is overconfident in

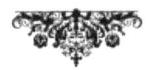

his/her skills. This may be a hard thing to spot-especially for learners who are new to the class-but if you don't ever find any signs of humility after attending few classes, start asking questions. And if you never ever hear "I don't know," or a similar response, be wary of the answers you receive from him/her. Nobody in this world knows everything. In fact, the belief that one knows everything makes it really hard to grow and learn-something that awesome teachers don't ever stop doing.

2. He makes the class about him. Talks more, listens less. Instead of helping you in cultivating your own practice he/she seems to be more interested in showing his/her own practice. Spends most of the time during the class in bragging about his great and famous teachers. Or maybe he/she continuously teaches poses that the class isn't ready for - just for the sake of feeding his/her ego.

3. He insists to practice a pose in a particular way - but can't explain any good reasons behind it. A pretty common answer or explanation is "Because I said so." As if you're a kid being guided by a nursery teacher. Yoga teachers shouldn't ask their

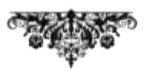

students to do anything in a particular way until they've a good and solid reason. And they must explain the reason behind any pose, sequence or any other technique if they're asked to do so.

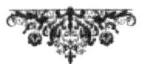

CHAPTER 27

YOUR PATH - AFTER YOU BECOME A YOGA TEACHE

Many Yoga teacher interns have different reasons why they seek out an initial 200 hour Level 1 training course. After teaching classes for a while, some experienced teachers are looking to teach students who have much in common with them. For example: The teacher who is very fit is often looking to teach students who are athletes.

In some cases, a doula, mid-wife, nurse, or a mother may be drawn to pre-natal Yoga. Teachers with young families, and children of their own, may be seeking to teach Yoga. A Yoga teacher, who is past the point of middle age, may be looking to teach students who have something in common with him or her.

Regardless of our personal reasons, each of us chooses a different path, and sometimes, that path may be one of specialization. In our first Yoga instructor training, we may have reflected upon the fact that there is a divine plan for each of us.

There are instances when our Yogic path is based upon finding a purpose, realization of a skill set, or our personal code of ethics. In order for us to choose the correct path, we have to look within ourselves, on a personal quest, to find a more fulfilling and focused direction.

At the same time, any direction we choose should not be an obsession of self-love or self-hate. Some of us whole-heartedly value the opinions of others. This can be a good thing, if the advice we receive is based on reality. The point being - in our lifetime, we will receive advice that is not in our best interest.

With that said - some opinions you hear may be in the best interest of the person giving you the information. For one reason, or another, some people give opinions, which tend to hold others back from making progress. While this is not always the case, we should always logically measure any advice.

HOW TO BECOME A CERTIFIED YOGA TEACHER WITHOUT LEAVING THE HOUSE

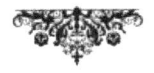

Yoga is a form of exercise that proves to be effective in cleansing the body, relaxing the mind and increasing the flexibility of the body. With this, many health problems can be addressed through yoga. This is why more and more people turn to yoga teachers to help them cure their health problems. Though there are many courses teaching you how to become a teacher, it is not possible for everyone to attend one. However, to be completely truthful teacher training has never been easier and here's why.

The internet has made it possible today for anyone to learn without having to leave the house. However, the main thing you have to remember before you practice at home is to first understand the practice. With the right postures, within your limitations, you will be able to avail of the full benefit of yoga, and pretty soon be able to teach yoga too.

There are many DVDs, books and internet sites teaching you about the various postures that benefit different health and cleansing problems. Once you choose the right book or DVD to learn yoga, get yourself a mat and unrestrictive

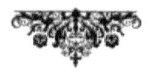

clothing. Dimming the lights and switching off phones can create the right atmosphere of peace for yoga.

It is possible to become a teacher only by practicing to perfection. So once you get the hang of the different yoga postures, practice till you can teach the postures to others without having to refer to any literature or DVD. Once this is attained, you can very well start your own yoga classes or join health classes and gyms to teach yoga to others.

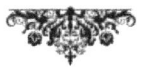

CHAPTER 28

YOGA TEACHER ETHICS AND GUIDELINES

Thee have been times when it has been stated that yoga teacher ethics were just a matter of common sense. Teachers have seen the looks in an intern's eyes, when the lecture starts. The intern's eyes tell me that he/she is thinking, "What's the big deal?" with respect to teacher ethics.

Yoga instructors are the guiding lights for all students interested in learning yogic methods. Teacher's operate under a series of ethics and moral guidelines. These guidelines are designed to help them teach yoga fairly, kindly, and morally. Yoga is a form of recreation guided by the key scriptures of kindness, compassion, generosity, tolerance, patience, helpfulness, forgiveness, and purity.

Walking the Talk

As a result, yoga instructors need to reflect these ethical stances in their teaching practice. A teacher may not constantly live up to these ideals in their day-to-day lives. Unfortunately, we are human and we make mistakes.

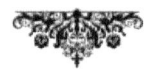

However, instructors must do whatever they can to promote these ideals through their teaching methods.

A good teacher understands that yoga is a noble path of life, with an extended history of highly successful teachers. They must align their behavior and their teachings with these teachers. Successfully promoting the values of yoga can help teachers reach their students on a deeper level, beyond the physical benefits of the postures.

For example, imagine you are a yoga student, and your teacher swears at you as you struggle with a Downward Dog Pose. His or her lack of patience will greatly disturb your mental well-being. It may even cause you to become resentful of your yoga teacher and to harbor feelings of anger, grief and angst.

A successful yoga instructor will tolerate the mistakes of others in the classroom. If a teacher must criticize a student, they should do it fairly. They should never make fun of the student or their attempts at practicing a yoga technique. Instead, they should gently focus on the facts and give solutions that help a student to learn. Whenever you spend time with a great teacher, you learn how to

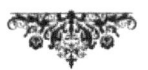

154

improve yourself, surpass an obstacle, or modify a technique.

How do we Apply Ethics in our Classes?

Yoga teacher's must also respect the physical "bubble" around their students. Slight, brief touches, are acceptable for correction purposes. The teacher must respect a student if they don't tolerate being touched in any way.

Yoga ethics demand that a teacher be truthful with his or her students. An instructor should never praise a student's progress falsely. Instead, he or she must be honest with the student about their technique. On the other hand, the teacher must be understanding, patient, and fair, with all students. Our students will be inspired to work harder by a teacher who shows compassion and honesty.

Teaching students fairness, compassion, and honesty is a big part of the reason why yoga teacher ethics are such a "big deal." The poses, breathing, and exercises of yoga are important, but are not the primary benefit of a practice. Instead, a yoga teacher is working to impart upon, his or her students, the morals and ethics that guide yoga as a practice.

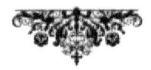

Yoga Teacher Ethics and Liability

Yoga is all about the mind and body connection. It is about being in tune with your breath and your posture, so the issue of ethics and liability is often far from many yoga instructors' minds. That is not to say these teachers are unethical, only that this indicates their passion for yoga. The fact is their students often take precedent over potential ethical and legal concerns.

Yoga is a physical, mental, emotional, and spiritual endeavor, and as such, any skilled yoga instructor must help guide students into the proper techniques in order to achieve the best results. During a posture (asana) practice, this often involves physical contact of various degrees. While touching may seem a benign endeavor, within the confines of a safe yoga studio, it very easily can turn into something questionable, even if performed with the best intentions. Therefore, it is imperative for any teacher to take the time to consider ethics and liability as it relates to their instruction.

Aside from the pragmatic use of physical touch to help align a student into a proper position, the human touch has an essential quality to it that, in a healing art such as yoga,

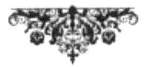

should be encouraged. That said, it is important to consider acceptable boundaries and the individual nature of people while discerning when, where, and how to touch someone.

Some teachers ask their students prior to instruction if they welcome touch, and if so, to what degree. Some students may prefer a hands-off approach, even when it comes to alignment; in which case, it would behoove both the yoga instructor and the student to be aware of such a boundary in advance. Other students may welcome touch and thrive on it. Of course, it goes without saying that touch, which could facilitate injury or be construed as sexually invasive, should always remain off limits regardless of the student.

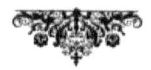

CHAPTER 29

YOGA TEACHER CERTIFICATION - YOUR UNTAPPED POTENTIAL

What is your untapped potential? Why do people take a certification course to become a Yoga teacher? Could Yoga teacher training help you to find inherent talents that have remained hidden inside you? Let's look at these, and many other questions, related to finding natural resources within each of us.

What is your untapped potential? Most of us let a few set backs in life guide us down a well-beaten path that is traveled by many. Most people do not consider their full potential. Instead, they become conditioned to settle for less from life. They "play it safe," and become extremely conscious of risk.

Your untapped potential is your ability that lies hidden in dormancy. You may not have had time to consider what you really want to do in life. Assessing your natural talents

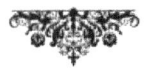

is a start, but envisioning where your natural talents could carry you is your untapped potential.

Why do people take a certification course to become a Yoga teacher? There are a wide variety of reasons why people take intensive courses. Some interns may feel a calling toward teaching Yoga as a vocation. Some choose to teach as a part-time hobby.

There are many, who take Yoga teacher courses, to help friends and family members. In this case, they are seeking enough information to teach safely. Rarely do interns have visions of a big Yoga teacher salary. It is possible to earn respectable wages, but this requires teachers to market themselves.

The marketing aspect tends to be a "turn off" for those who do not seek full time employment. This runs parallel to the mindset of many artists and writers, who begin to realize that a successful marketing campaign may require 50%, or more, of their time.

Could Yoga teacher training help you to find inherent talents that have remained hidden inside you? Yes, a Yoga teacher intensive course makes it possible to tap into the

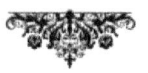

inner-self through self-realization. For anyone who experiences this awakening of consciousness, the world around them has changed.

This change is due to a transformation from within. At this point it is up to each individual, as to what he or she will do with complete awareness. A few may use it to garner a respectable Yoga instructor salary, while most will use the information they learn to help others.

Untapped potential means many things to different people, but it usually comes down to our personal values. Within each of us, what we see as valuable will be different. Regardless of our differences, a Yoga teacher intensive will guide us to find our true purpose in life.

MAKING YOUR MARK IN THE YOGA PROFESSION

If you have decided to take your love for yoga to the next step by becoming a certified instructor, you need to know what it takes to build your reputation in the industry. You can become the instructor that everyone wants to sit under by investing in yourself and being dedicated to your teaching. If you have a strong passion and knowledge, you

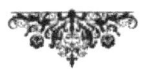

need to find out where to get classes to become a yoga instructor so that you can make your mark in this fast growing profession. There are steps that can help you to build a solid teaching foundation.

Identify your area of interest

The first thing you need to do is to establish what you are good at or where your talents lie. This knowledge will allow you to narrow your focus and to select the best courses. You should ask yourself questions like what your favorite style of yoga is and why. When you know your favorite type of yoga, you can determine your niche market.

Create an online presence

Having an online presence is essential in the world today. If you want to reach a wide audience without spending money, you need to be on social media. It also helps to have a website that will allow you to include more information about your studio. An active blog page is a great way to communicate with current and potential students on a regular basis as you can post articles about your favorite activity.

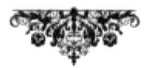

Offer Private Sessions

While the ideal situation is teaching a live class, in a world where people are busy and have no time to schedule classes, offering private or personal sessions can be a way to attract students from everywhere. You can offer the classes in person or online where you can teach the class through online technology like chat sites. You can also use videos to reach students who may not be close to your location.

Create a fun atmosphere

The days are gone where people associated yoga with a serious atmosphere, where everyone just hummed with a serious look on their face. Today, you can get the experience you need while having fun at it. By ensuring that your students enjoy the classes, you can make a name for yourself, as you will attract more students. You can organize a yoga retreat every few months to help your student's enjoy the experience.

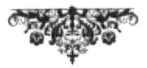

CHAPTER 30

TEN REASONS TO BECOME A YOGA TEACHER

Having a healthy lifestyle is necessary. If you are interested in living a healthy lifestyle, then you might want to consider taking up a yoga class. A lot of people have admitted that this discipline have changed them a lot, not only physically but also in terms of other aspects such as the mental and spiritual aspect.

People who have been practicing this discipline for a number of year's have considered moving up to the next level and become an instructor. Apparently, these numbers of people who have taken an interest in this practice are gradually increasing, that is why, the number of yoga schools providing teaching certificate programs are also increasing.

Becoming an instructor of yoga is a rewarding job, not because it guarantees you with a lot of earnings but because it lets you enjoy what you are doing while also keeping your body in a healthy state. Instead of having to

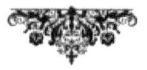

think it over, here are ten reasons to become a yoga teacher.

Teaching this practice can serve as a compensating part time job. We are all aware that our economy is shaky and having an additional source of income would be a great way to meet the ends. If you decide to teach yoga, you'd be able to earn an additional compensation while also enjoying the hobby that you like the best. Teaching yoga can be a great way for long time yoga practitioners to earn while also being able to practice yoga.

You are able to share your perspectives in life to others through yoga. Through becoming a yoga instructor, you are able to share your views in life to other people. Advance your knowledge and skills in yoga. If you are going to take the certification program for yoga instructors, you will be able to enhance your skills and knowledge in yoga.

Share your knowledge about yoga to other people. Through enrolling to a certification program, you will be able to share your knowledge about yoga formally and in a professional way. Yoga instructors can inspire people to

learn yoga. You can become an inspiration to others to practice yoga if you become an effective instructor of this yoga.

Maintain a healthy lifestyle. While you consider teaching this practice as a part time job or additional source of income, you can still maintain a healthy lifestyle through this profession.

Become physically fit. This is one of the benefits of yoga, and while you are considering this as a job, you are also able to get the benefits of practicing yoga.

Become well known in the field of yoga. If you put your heart in teaching you will definitely be able to build your own name in the industry.

Make necessary changes to your lifestyle. Teaching yoga can be a lifestyle changing decision. Although you've been practicing yoga for a long time already, teaching yoga will open new doors to you, if you've been just practicing before, after becoming an instructor, you will have to exert extra effort and do well in your every class.

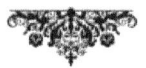

USE YOUR FREE FIRST CLASS THE RIGHT WAY TO GROW YOUR YOGA BUSINESS

Many yoga business offering free first classes, getting students in the door through this promotion, and then leaving it up to the students to figure out for themselves what they're supposed to get out the whole darn experience. Here's some insight: most students leave the yoga studio bewildered, overwhelmed, possibly in pain, exhausted and sweaty. Beginner yoga students especially feel the wrath, but experienced students in a new environment can easily feel this way too. Would you want to come back for more of that?

Of course we all know that if they just kept it up, after even a few classes they would start to feel more relaxed, welcome, and in tune with their bodies in a way never experienced before. But go tell that to them. No, really...go tell that to them!

The first class a student takes at your yoga studio will often make or break whether they come back, or even stick to yoga at all. And getting a student to come back is imperative to your yoga business. So, it stands to reason

166

then that this class is the most important class they will ever take with you. Why aren't you paying more attention to it? It's your opportunity to introduce your philosophy, your ambiance, and your teaching style to them. It's your opportunity to make them feel special, invited, and a valued participant and member of your community. And its your opportunity - and more importantly your responsibility - to find out why they came to yoga in the first place, and inform them on why your yoga studio is the best one to help them accomplish their goals.

So let me ask you:

- Who is the first person to greet your new student?
- What is being told to the new student?
- Are they shown around and made comfortable, or are they met with indifference?
- Do they know what to expect out of the class? (I.e. that they will probably be a little uncomfortable, a little overwhelmed, and a litle sweaty - but that they also will experience amazing results after just another class or two?)
- Does the teacher learn their name, and use it during class?

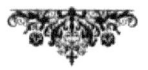

- Do you ask them questions about why they started yoga, what they hope to get out of it, what their concerns are? (Let me tell you what this is NOT - it is not saying - "do you have any questions?" Most beginners don't even know what they don't know. Help them out!)

The first class a new student takes is the catalyst for all future interaction - for the possibility of a long-term realtionship - with this student. From a profit standpoint, each new student could be worth thousands of dollars to you in your yoga business. This isn't just a willy-nilly chance for them to 'try that yoga thing,' and for you to cross your fingers and pray to Buddha that they come back. You have to view it as a business meeting with one of the most profitable potential clients, and treat it with great respect. Because what's at stake is your yoga business growth, your opportunity to transform more lives, and their journey on a yogic path. No small thing, but it only requires a different perspective on your part and a little extra effort. It's worth it.

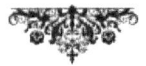

CHAPTER 31

YOGA MYTH - YOGA IS NOT A SPIRITUAL
PRACTICE

It is true that there are some Hatha classes, which resemble "exercise classes." There has been some mixing of Pilates and Yoga, within the past two decades. In the West, some styles of Hatha Yoga, teach very little about Pranayama, Mantra, Japa, Mudras, Bandhas, Meditation, Shatkarmas, Doshas, the Subtle Body, the History of Yoga, or Yogic Philosophy.

As a result, some Yoga classes have become more like calisthenics classes. So, why has Yoga changed so much, when it left India? Why is the practice of Bhakti so popular in India, and is scarcely known in the West?

Quite simply, Yoga has transcended cultures, and it is going through another evolutionary phase. Many people "try" Yoga, but the serious practitioner continues to practice for decades. A Yogi, or Yogini, has decided to continue his or her practice for life, because of the benefits.

169

When we are young, we experience the physical aspects of life to their fullest potential. We challenge our bodies to their limits. No matter what age we are, being physically aware of our bodies, comes first. This same awareness happens in a class.

For most of us, the mental, emotional, and spiritual, planes of existence are developed as we age. The same is true within Yoga practice. As we continue to practice, and the year's go by, we begin to realize the many benefits, which are not physical.

If we practice Yoga for decades, we are at peace with ourselves and our surroundings. The many benefits of Yoga are not visible to the human eye. If a person has stress under control, good health, peace of mind, self-confidence, or a stronger relationship with God, we cannot detect it at a glance, and that is the deception, which most people make.

Yoga has so many benefits, which a superficial person would miss. If you want instant results, you will not have the patience to practice for years. The impatient person,

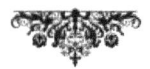

who is quick to judge everything, and wants to instantly lose weight, should find a liposuction surgeon. The mental, emotional, and spiritual aspects of Yoga will be missed, but this person would not appreciate them anyway.

Getting back to the spiritual aspect - It is part of the Yogic package; if you continue to practice Yoga - spiritual health will reveal itself to you in the form of the religion you are most comfortable with. For those who say spiritual health is a bad thing, I am sorry they have tunnel vision. It is a shame, when people cannot live in harmony with other people and the world around them.

YOGA TEACHER LIABILITY INSURANCE

After an intern has successfully completed a Yoga teacher training course, he or she is looking for teaching positions and considering many side issues. One of the main issues is liability insurance. Below is a question and answer session regarding Yoga teachers and liability insurance.

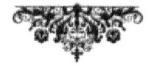

Q. What if a student did not indicate a specific health issue and has a problem, ailment, or physical condition that I am unaware of?

A: You cannot read minds, but you can develop a preliminary questionnaire for all of your students to answer, before they enter your classes. A detailed questionnaire makes you aware of their ailments and limitations. For Yoga teachers, negligence is when we take risks with our student's health and well being.

Negligence also happens when we know of a pre-existing problem, but we fail to take action, by creating a safe environment and practice for our students. If a student does not tell you about his or her pre-existing health conditions, when you have an established track record of establishing student safety policies, you cannot be held responsible for a student's actions.

Q. Likewise, what if a student indicates a pre-existing condition and then does not follow teacher safety guidelines and corresponding information for student safety?

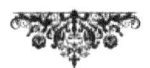

A: You should continually mention safety precautions during your classes. Sometimes, a stubborn student may have to be warned or advised to stop practicing in your Yoga classes. If a student is taking risks against your advice, you should address this directly. You are not responsible for students who do not follow your advice in regard to their safety.

Q. How do teachers protect themselves from being the subjects of lawsuits?

A: Firstly, anyone can be sued for anything. It's a matter of whether a judge feels a case has legitimacy. A small number of Yoga teachers could find themselves at risk for accusations regarding negligence, lack of ethics, or harassment lawsuits. However, there are very few Yoga students who have ever complained about negligence, ethics violations, or harassment.

This is one more reason why certified Yoga teachers should be active in their continuing education. As long as you have a track record of professional behavior, establishing safety guidelines, giving modifications, watching your class, and building a rapport with students,

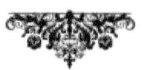

you should be fine. Giving an extra safety tip, making handouts available, or mentioning a specific contraindication, during your classes, establishes a history of your deep concern over student safety.

Q. What are your thoughts about Yoga teachers acquiring liability insurance?

A: Most Yoga teachers have liability insurance for themselves or the entire staff at the center. Teachers should consider Yoga or sports liability insurance, depending upon the reputation of the company and the rates. Most teachers admit, they never had to use it; but liability insurance gives each teacher a "safety net." You never really know if any insurance is good until you have a problem.

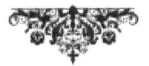

CHAPTER 32

YOGA FOR THE ELDERLY

Growing old is also the time when you are more susceptible to some ailments. This makes the application of yoga for the elderly even more important. The best of all the good qualities of yoga for the elderly is the chanting of Om at the end of every class.

To do so, senior's should realize that practicing Yoga for the elderly takes into account gradualism. My special interest is Yoga for the elderly and for arthritis sufferers. Yoga for the elderly can improve circulation and minimize arthritis and digestive disorders caused by inactivity. More interesting than Yoga for the Elderly, sure, but I'm not technical.

Elderly

The elderly had my special interest because my own parents and my mother-in-law are becoming older. The proportion of elderly people in our society is increasing, and will increase even more in the next decade. There are several reasons why it is so important to teach yoga to elderly people.

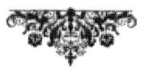

There are some general precautions to keep in mind when teaching yoga to elderly people. Teaching yoga to the elderly has enriched me very much. One other aspect that makes me feel privileged to be teaching the elderly is their surrender during relaxation, and even more during the deep final relaxation (yoga nidra).

Exercise

These recommendations further suggest that combinations of moderate and vigorous exercise can be used to meet the requirements and that bouts of moderate-intensity exercise lasting a minimum of 10 minutes can be accumulated to achieve the 30 minute minimum. Yoga is a safe, inexpensive, non-impact form of exercise that improves cardiovascular health.

Breathing

Yoga practice, which involves rhythmic stretching movements and breathing, may help improve and stabilize mood. Spend a few moments of quiet here, listening to your breathing and clearing your mind. Thus, a 30 min program of yogic stretch and breathing exercises which is simple to learn and which can be practised even by the

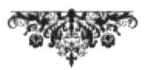

elderly had a markedly 'invigorating' effect on perceptions of both mental and physical energy and increased high positive mood.

This position also normalizes blood pressure and breathing, thus providing many benefits to asthma and heart patients. Yoga is a complete science, focusing on the breathing movement, posture and meditation. Deep and controlled breathing will help any elder face the problems of old age with a more positive and relaxed attitude. You might be wondering why such a simple and common thing like breathing can become an element which can make the difference in a yoga session.

WHY DO SOME RELIGIOUS FUNDAMENTALISTS FEAR YOGA?

For many non-practitioners of Yoga, it is Intolerance for something they do not understand. This seems harmless at first, but cries of witchcraft are never a good omen. However, every method of healing has its critics.

Yoga has also been accused of being a "launching point" to export Hinduism. This is very interesting, considering

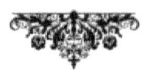

the large numbers of Yoga practitioners who are not Hindus. Some Yogis and Yoginis do convert to Hinduism, but the "calling" had to come from within themselves. Within North America, most Yoga teachers are not Hindus at all and I have yet to witness religious conversion in progress.

For fundamentalist Hindus that believe Yoga and Hinduism cannot be separate, sorry to break the news, but it has already happened. Yoga was interpreted in many ways by a variety of cultures and partial facets of Yoga have grown independently. Some Hatha Yoga styles do not even practice meditation.

Yoga students outside India, pick and choose what they want to learn from Yoga. At this time, physical mastery seems to be most popular. This is why Yoga teachers outside India focus primarily on physical health. Many western students think only of Hatha Yoga, when they hear the word "Yoga."

This is why Yoga cannot really be controlled, regulated, or patented. How do you control people's thoughts,

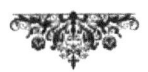

actions, physical practice, prayers, meditation, or songs? The whole concept of controlling Yoga is ludicrous.

Fundamentalists of different religions work together, quite by accident, to divide the world's religions into mobs of intolerance. Their real fear is loss of control. So they speak in "absolutes." For example: "You will burn in hell, if you do not, do as I say" and "All of the non-believers are going to Hell."

The real problem with Yoga, for the fundamentalist of any religion, is that it can be practiced by anyone from any religion. Yoga is not exclusive: The laws are universal and interchangeable with every religion. This allows a Yoga practitioner to work independently on his or her spiritual health and work toward enlightenment.

What is wrong with working toward the common good? The idea of working toward enlightenment and self-perfection are considered blasphemy to some. However, can you imagine a world where men and women did not try to improve themselves?

The objectives of Yoga are complete heath, self-improvement, self realization, and tranquility. With these

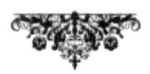

benefits acquired any Yoga practitioner can help others and work for the common good.

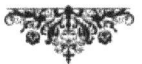

CHAPTER 33

WHAT TO LOOK FOR IN A GOOD YOGA TEACHER

A good yoga teacher should primarily be someone who inspires you to practice and to better yourself. Yoga is ultimately about bringing peace to yourself and the teacher's teachings should encourage this in you.

A good yoga teacher should be someone with a lot of enthusiasm for yoga, that is someone who enjoys not only practising and learning yoga themselves, but also someone who enjoys teaching yoga too.

The ultimate goal of yoga is to bring peace into oneself and to transmit this sense of peace to others. Of course yoga is a path. In our human world we can only strive to be peaceful. However the goal should be there. Hence a good yoga teacher should be one whose goal it is to be peaceful and also one who has an understanding of what peace or shanti actually is.The ancient Indian scriptures talk a lot about 'shanti' or peace. Shanti according to the scriptures is the original nature of the soul. There are also a lot of teachings that talk about the seventh chakra as

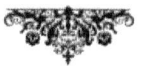

181

being a place where peace can be experienced. Also the teachings of 'ahimsa' or non-violence talk about peaceful conduct. A good yoga teacher should have a good understanding of this.

In addition to this a good yoga teacher should have a good understanding that yoga is not just asana or physical practice but is something much deeper. The teacher should be one who always encourages you to focus your awareness on your breath in order to bring you into a state of meditation. The good should always be aware of the ashtanga or eight limbs of yoga which include rules for social and moral conduct, meditation, breath control and so forth. The good teacher, however, should still have an understanding of asana and anatomy in order to correct the physical posture. The eight limbs of yoga do include asana or physical practice too.

The teacher should understand that yoga is about health. As yoga has developed many people have become aware of the health benefits of yoga practice (including those of meditation) and the good teacher should understand and teach this. Following a sattvic or pure diet is an important step in yoga. It is useful when following a pure diet to eat

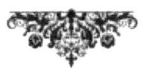

organic foods that contain no pesticides and are grown in a manner designed to keep the soil fertile and the products full of nutrients. The good teacher should guide you with good diet and good health.

The good teacher encourages you not to be competitive but to work on yourself. He or she understands that everyone is different, has different genetics and that everyone comes to yoga with their own needs. A sign of a good teacher is that he or she tells you not to look at others during the class. This helps you focus on yourself and your own development and this should ideally what the good teacher leads you towards.

The good teacher gives good adjustments but does not push you too much. He or she rather encourages you, helps you to see your potential and guides you towards a point of peace within yourself.

The good teacher has a strong desire to help you with your journey and to guide you towards peace.

The good teacher likes all aspects of yoga. This includes chanting, breathing techniques, meditation, philosophy.

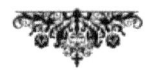

He or she sees all the benefits of the different branches of yoga and helps you with those that appeal to you.

Above all the good yoga teacher is someone you can bond with and form a relationship with. He or she should be someone who you can relate to, someone who is on the same path as you and someone who encourages you to follow your path.

QUALITIES OF A GOOD YOGA TEACHER

There are many qualities that define a good Yoga teacher. The following highlight some of these qualities:

Presence

A good yoga teacher is one that commands attention. This is felt when the teacher walks into the training room. The teacher radiates energy that makes the student want to practice yoga even when they are feeling down as he or she should make you feel at ease and welcome thereby lifting the student's spirit.

Physical Skills

The yoga teacher should possess the skills that he or she is trying to impart on the students. It is easy for one to

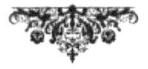

teach what one knows and practices as opposed to what one does not know.

Personalization

A good yoga teacher ought to possess a signature sequence or a trademark sequence. This should be real and original and the yoga instructor has to own it. The teacher should possess the ability to turn a complex situation into a simple situation that can be achieved by anyone and everyone.

Versatility

The teacher should be in tune with the needs of his or her students and should be flexible enough to adjust the training to address the requirements of the students, without compromising the training requirements of the class. He should have the ability to connect with the spirituality of the students without undermining the subject matter of the class and should be able go out of his or her way to meet the requirements of the students.

Keen to Details

Yoga teaches that God is in details therefore a good yoga training session flourishes in details. Observing details,

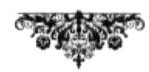

even while doing your own practice is what will heighten your experience therefore a good teacher will be keen to always ensure that the student's are doing the poses in the right way. This shows commitment to the job.

Language

The language used should be a common language understood by all. Every word spoken by the yoga teacher should count and should serve the purpose of the training thus meeting the set goals.

Clear Instructions with Room to Breathe

The students should be able to understand the instructions given to them by their teacher. The instructions should be clear, concise and easy to follow. There should be room to breathe in between the paces to allow the student to feel and explore themselves.

Punctual

The teacher should always be on time in beginning and ending his or her classes as the students also have other schedules of their own.

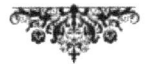

CONCLUSION

How many of your students told you that they attended classes to improve their personalities? Just a quick guess: None of your students considered Yoga for improving their personality. Yet, personality improvement is a by-product of a sense of awareness. Yoga practitioners learn to become conscious of their thoughts, words, and actions.

Anyone who practices any form of Yoga, on a regular basis, knows that the results go much further than longer, leaner muscles and greater flexibility. The breathing and meditative portions of a daily Yogic lifestyle can bring peace and understanding to the mind. Pranayama and meditation can teach one how to cope with daily stress and anxiety, while learning how to find overall peace within one's self. The breathing techniques, alone, can be an extremely useful tool to apply in all aspects of life.

Personality Development for Young People

Yoga can also help young people develop and grow positive personality traits. Meditation and Yoga encourage inner reflection by sitting quietly, tuning out extra stimulation, noise, and negative thoughts. This

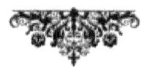

promotes the ability to learn who you are, what makes you happy, what makes you uneasy, and what is important in your life. Sometimes, life gets too busy, which causes impressionable young people to go with the flow of a group, instead of thinking about the long-term consequences. Yoga gives people, of all ages, the time to truly reflect, and make choices based on their own thoughts and feelings, rather than others'.

Gratitude

Yoga instills a desire and ability to feel gratitude for life. Through steady practice, young people learn to be mindful of each moment. They learn to appreciate all of the small things that happen during each moment. Perhaps it is a smile from a friend or the beauty of a wildflower. When young people learn to be grateful for the things in their lives, the little stresses and annoyances of daily life become less important. When you do not allow yourself to place importance on unimportant things, you become more grateful for those things that truly do matter.

Accountability

Many young people, today, are not made to feel accountable for their actions, thoughts, or feelings.

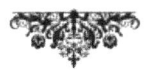

Sometimes, parents are making excuses for their children or getting them out of binds, without asking the child to take responsibility. Yoga and meditation can help young kids realize that they, alone, are responsible for their actions, and how they act, affects how others perceive them.

Inner Peace

As youngsters struggle to find out who they are, the road can sometimes be rocky and full of twists and turns. Pranayama and meditation allow young people an outlet to find an inner sense of calm and peace. When a youngster possesses this important inner peace, others can easily recognize it. An inner peace allows you to make the best choices in life.

As teachers, we should encourage our students to understand themselves based on their internal reference points rather than those of the external world. This practice will inflect our teaching in both practical and subtle ways.

To guide others is an art of infinite subtlety, although it is rarely appreciated as such. As our understanding and command of the art of teaching develops, so will the well-

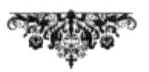

being of our students. Deepening that understanding means recognizing that all of our instruction and guidance must rest on a particular foundation: to help our students become "internally referential."

We understand who we are based on our perceptions of the world around us. We learn to compare ourselves with others and value ourselves in accordance with how we stack up with them. Through this process, we become "externally referential"-we make sense of ourselves by referring to outer standards. By the time we become adults, our self-conceptions are largely borrowed from what we have been told by our parents, family members, friends, teachers, and the commercial media. We do things to look good or be popular, not necessarily because they are our soul's desire or our life's true purpose. Compounding the problem, advertisers incessantly bombard us with messages saying, at root, "You are falling short when compared to others. You had better buy your way out of this embarrassing situation."

Defining ourselves in terms of external references is a dead end because it means ignoring the desires of the soul. As yoga teachers, we must work to help our student's

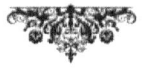

understand this. In fact, one of our main jobs is to shift the paradigm of external reference to one of internal reference. Our work is to help our students-particularly beginners-become aware of who they are as distinct from what they have been told they are. One way to do this is by defying common practice and not telling our students what they are. Instead of placing them in categories and destroying their uniqueness with labels, we can tell our students what they can do to change, grow, and find themselves.

Becoming a Yoga teacher can be a rewarding career in all aspects. You can help impart knowledge that will help develop inner strength and well being of your students. But before making that crucial decision about becoming a Yoga instructor, there are a few things which you must consider.

Since you will need to teach people, you need to access the needs of the environment you reside in and determine if there is demand for Yoga lessons. You can also search the web for Yoga schools in your surrounding and also in hotels and fitness centers to determine the level of employment for any Yoga professional.

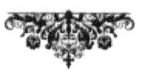

After ascertaining that there is demand, you will require the necessary certifications to enable you deliver better services to your clients and students. Although you can start teaching Yoga before getting the certifications, it's imperative that you get certified. This will require that you master the theory part of it and teach a class of students while being supervised to ensure that you attain the necessary certifications. It's imperative that you master the general concepts that will enable you teach any type of Yoga and also cultivate a culture that will enable you make it part and parcel of your life.

Ensure that your students take a process at a time as they may get injured if you make a rush switch from one program to another. Ensure that you have enough confidence by practicing with your family members before you deal with your students.